W9-BMH-180

WINNER!
WINNER!
300
CALORIE
DINNERS!

Publications International, Ltd.

Some of the products listed in this publication may be in limited distribution.

Pictured on the front cover (*clockwise from top left*): Mu Shu Turkey (*page 62*), Red Wine & Oregano Beef Kabobs (*page 74*), Turkey Sausage & Spinach Stuffed Shells (*page 60*), Veggie Tostadas (*page 108*), Mini Meatloaves (*page 78*), Veggie Pizza Pitas (*page 38*), Turkey Sliders (*page 44*), and Kale & Mushroom Stuffed Chicken Breasts (*page 56*).

Pictured on the back cover (*from left to right*): Garlic Pork with Roasted Red Potatoes (*page 68*), Turkey & Veggie Roll-Ups (*page 54*), and Artichoke and Tomato Pasta (*page 40*).

ISBN: 978-1-64030-499-4

Manufactured in China.

8 7 6 5 4 3 2 1

Nutritional Analysis: Every effort has been made to check the accuracy of the nutritional information that appears with each recipe. However, because numerous variables account for a wide range of values for certain foods, nutritive analyses in this book should be considered approximate. Different results may be obtained by using different nutrient databases and different brand-name products.

Microwave Cooking: Microwave ovens vary in wattage. Use the cooking times as guidelines and check for doneness before adding more time.

Note: This book is for informational purposes and is not intended to provide medical advice. Neither Publications International, Ltd., nor the authors, editors or publisher takes responsibility for any possible consequences from any treatment, procedure, exercise, dietary modification, action, or applications of medication or preparation by any person reading or following the information in this cookbook. The publication of this book does not constitute the practice of medicine, and this cookbook does not replace your physician, pharmacist or health-care specialist. **Before undertaking any course of treatment or nutritional plan, the authors, editors and publisher advise the reader to check with a physician or other health-care provider.**

WARNING: Food preparation, baking and cooking involve inherent dangers: misuse of electric products, sharp electric tools, boiling water, hot stoves, allergic reactions, foodborne illnesses and the like, pose numerous potential risks. Publications International, Ltd. (PIL) assumes no responsibility or liability for any damages you may experience as a result of following recipes, instructions, tips or advice in this publication.

While we hope this publication helps you find new ways to eat delicious foods, you may not always achieve the results desired due to variations in ingredients, cooking temperatures, typos, errors, omissions, or individual cooking abilities.

TABLE OF CONTENTS

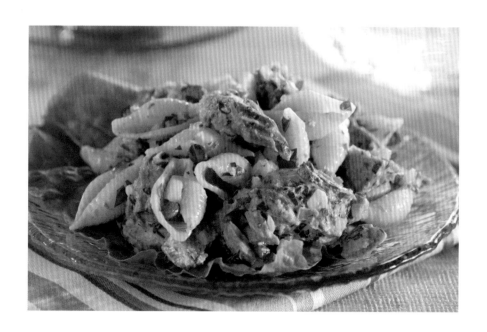

MAIN DISH SALADS

Garlic Bread and Salmon Salad

2 slices day-old light whole wheat bread
1 clove garlic, cut in half
7½ ounces canned, pouch or cooked salmon, flaked
½ cup chopped green onions, green parts only
1 cup cherry or grape tomatoes, halved
1 teaspoon olive oil
5 teaspoons white wine vinegar
1 tablespoon tomato juice
¼ teaspoon salt
¼ teaspoon black pepper
2 tablespoons minced fresh basil

1 Preheat broiler. Set rack 3 to 4 inches from heat. Rub one side of each bread slice with garlic. Discard garlic. Set bread, garlic side up, on broiler rack. Broil 20 to 30 seconds or until lightly browned; watch carefully and remove when done to avoid burning.

2 Set bread aside. When cool enough to handle, cut into 1-inch pieces.

3 Combine salmon, green onions and tomatoes in large serving bowl. Combine oil, vinegar, tomato juice, salt and pepper in cup. Pour over salmon mixture. Add garlic bread cubes and toss again. Sprinkle with basil.

Makes 4 servings (1 cup per serving)

nutrients per serving

Calories 123   **Total Fat** 4g   **Sodium** 430mg
Protein 15g   **Saturated Fat** 1g   **Fiber** 2g
Carbohydrate 8g **Cholesterol** 44mg

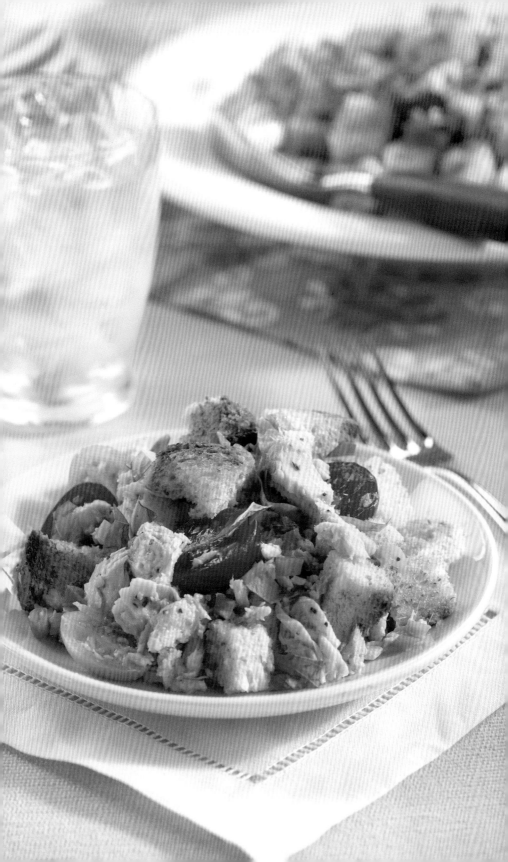

Mandarin Chicken Salad

3½ ounces thin rice noodles (rice vermicelli)
1 can (6 ounces) mandarin orange segments, chilled
⅓ cup honey
2 tablespoons rice wine vinegar
2 tablespoons reduced-sodium soy sauce
1 can (8 ounces) sliced water chestnuts, drained
4 cups shredded napa cabbage
1 cup shredded red cabbage
½ cup sliced radishes
4 thin slices red onion, cut in half and separated
3 boneless skinless chicken breasts (about 12 ounces), cooked and
    cut into strips

1 Place rice noodles in large bowl. Cover with hot water; soak 20 minutes or until soft. Drain.

2 Drain mandarin orange segments, reserving ⅓ cup liquid. Whisk reserved liquid, honey, vinegar and soy sauce in medium bowl. Add water chestnuts.

3 Divide noodles, cabbages, radishes and onion evenly among four serving plates. Top with chicken and orange segments. Remove water chestnuts from dressing and arrange on salads. Serve with remaining dressing.

Makes 4 servings

nutrients per serving

Calories 258
Protein 16g
Carbohydrate 46g
Total Fat 2g
Saturated Fat 1g
Cholesterol 34mg
Sodium 318mg
Fiber 2g

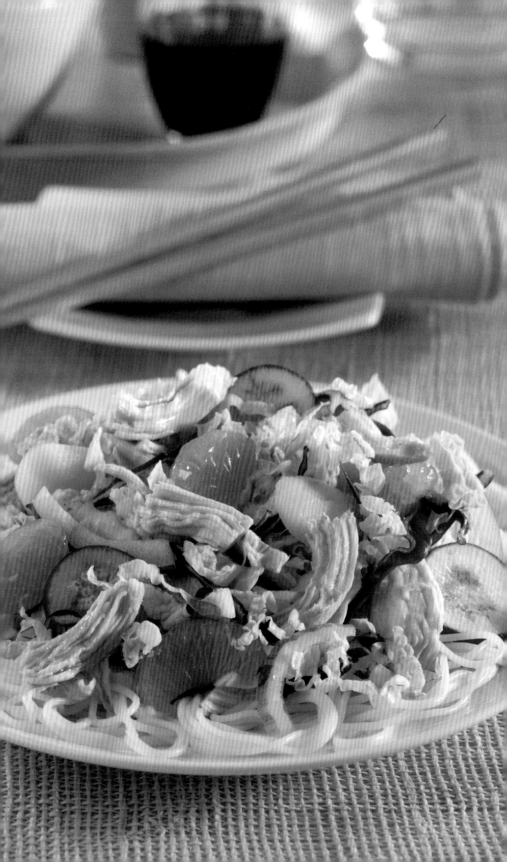

Thai Beef Salad

8 ounces beef flank steak
¼ cup soy sauce
2 jalapeño peppers,* finely chopped
2 tablespoons packed brown sugar
1 clove garlic, minced
½ cup lime juice
6 green onions, thinly sliced
4 carrots, diagonally cut into thin slices
½ cup finely chopped fresh cilantro
    Lettuce leaves

*Jalapeño peppers can sting and irritate the skin, so wear rubber gloves when handling peppers and do not touch your eyes.

1 Place flank steak in resealable food storage bag. Combine soy sauce, jalapeños, brown sugar and garlic in small bowl; pour over flank steak. Seal bag; turn to coat. Marinate in refrigerator for 2 hours.

2 Preheat broiler. Drain steak, discarding marinade. Place steak on rack of broiler pan. Broil 4 inches from heat 13 to 18 minutes for medium or to desired doneness, turning once. Remove from heat; let stand 15 minutes.

3 Thinly slice steak across grain. Toss with lime juice, green onions, carrots and cilantro in large bowl. Serve salad immediately over lettuce leaves.

Makes 4 servings (1 cup salad and 1 lettuce leaf per serving)

nutrients per serving

Calories 141	**Total Fat** 4g	**Sodium** 238mg
Protein 13g	**Saturated Fat** 2g	**Fiber** 3g
Carbohydrate 14g	**Cholesterol** 27mg	

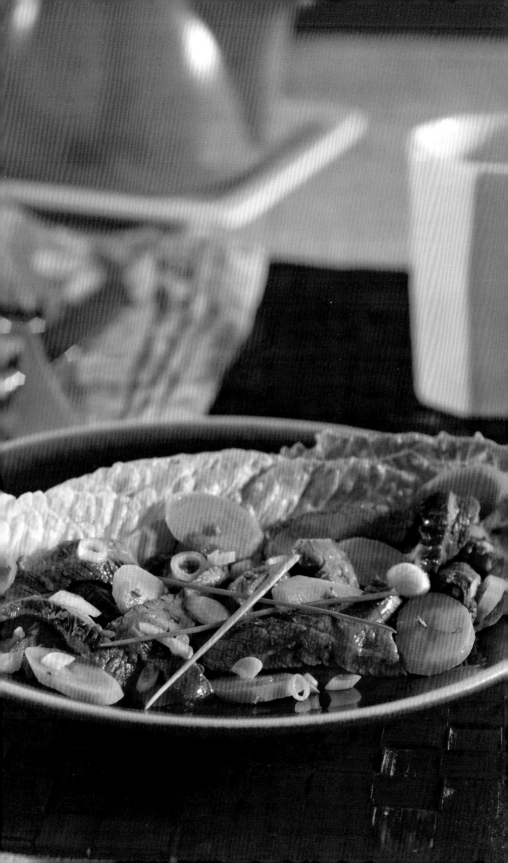

Leftover Turkey Caesar Salad with Homemade Croutons

4 slices (1 ounce each) whole grain bread, cut into ½-inch cubes
1 tablespoon olive oil
¼ teaspoon salt
¼ teaspoon dried basil
¼ teaspoon dried rosemary
¼ teaspoon dried thyme
6 cups chopped romaine lettuce
2 cups chopped cooked turkey breast
¼ cup shredded Parmesan cheese
¼ cup light Caesar salad dressing

1 Preheat oven to 375°F. Combine bread cubes, oil, salt, basil, rosemary and thyme on large baking sheet; gently toss to coat. Arrange in single layer. Bake 12 minutes, stirring halfway through. Cool completely.

2 Arrange lettuce on four serving plates. Top evenly with turkey, croutons and cheese; drizzle with dressing. Serve immediately.

Makes 4 servings

nutrients per serving

Calories 196   **Total Fat** 5g   **Sodium** 423mg
Protein 22g   **Saturated Fat** 2g   **Fiber** 5g
Carbohydrate 22g   **Cholesterol** 54mg

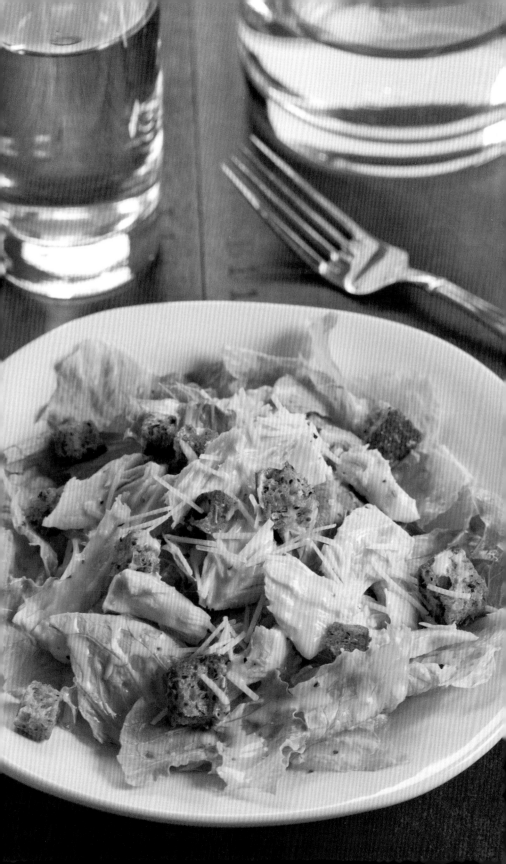

Wild Rice and Mixed Greens Salad

4 cups mixed baby greens

3 ounces baked or poached salmon, boneless skinless chicken breast *or*
white fish fillet

⅓ cup cooked brown and wild rice mixture*

2 tablespoons reduced-fat salad dressing

*Cook rice in fat-free reduced-sodium chicken broth for even more flavor.

1 Arrange greens on serving plate. Top with salmon.

2 Sprinkle rice mixture over salmon and greens. Drizzle with dressing.

Makes 1 serving

nutrients per serving

Calories 279	**Total Fat** 5g	**Sodium** 361mg
Protein 31g	**Saturated Fat** 1g	**Fiber** 6g
Carbohydrate 27g	**Cholesterol** 72mg	

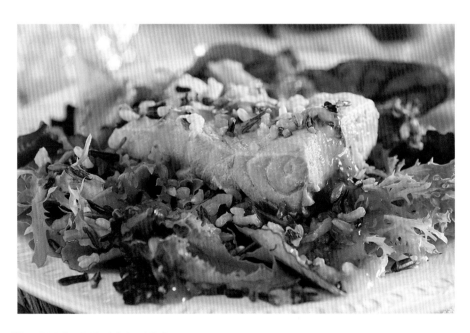

Salmon Pasta Salad

1 cup cooked medium pasta shells
1 can (about 6 ounces) canned red salmon, drained
½ cup finely chopped celery
2 tablespoons finely chopped red bell pepper
2 tablespoons chopped fresh parsley
2 tablespoons fat-free mayonnaise
1 green onion, finely chopped
1 tablespoon lemon juice
2 teaspoons capers
⅛ teaspoon paprika

Combine all ingredients in medium bowl. Cover; refrigerate until ready to serve.

Makes 2 servings (1½ cups per serving)

nutrients per serving

Calories 262
Protein 18g
Carbohydrate 26g

Total Fat 9g
Saturated Fat 2g
Cholesterol 21mg

Sodium 527mg
Fiber 2g

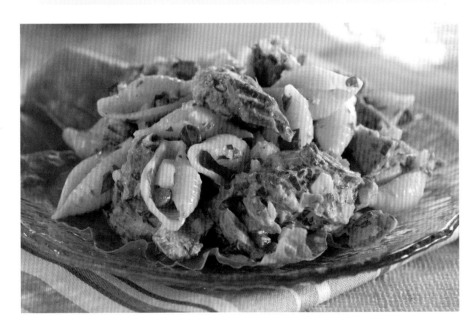

Chicken and Apple Spring Greens with Poppy Seeds

1 package (5 ounces) spring salad greens
12 ounces cooked chicken strips
1 large Golden Delicious apple, thinly sliced
⅓ cup thinly sliced red onion
1 ounce crumbled goat cheese (optional)
¼ cup cider vinegar
2 tablespoons sugar substitute
2 tablespoons canola oil
½ teaspoon poppy seeds
¼ teaspoon salt
⅛ teaspoon red pepper flakes

1 Arrange equal amounts greens, chicken, apple and onion on four plates. Sprinkle with cheese, if desired.

2 Combine vinegar, sugar substitute, oil, poppy seeds, salt and pepper flakes in small jar with tight-fitting lid; shake well. Drizzle dressing over salads.

Makes 4 servings

nutrients per serving

Calories 166	**Total Fat** 4g	**Sodium** 221mg
Protein 17g	**Saturated Fat** 1g	**Fiber** 4g
Carbohydrate 17g	**Cholesterol** 17mg	

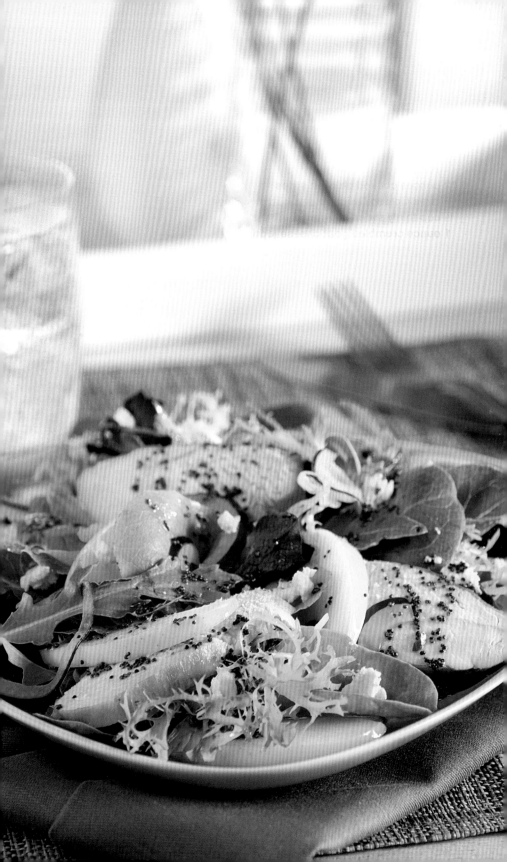

Chicken Caesar Salad with Homemade Croutons

3 to 4 slices (¾-inch-thick) whole grain artisan bread, cut into ¾-inch
    cubes (about 2 cups)
2 tablespoons olive oil
1½ teaspoons salt-free garlic-herb seasoning, divided
2 boneless skinless chicken breasts (about 4 ounces each)
8 cups torn romaine lettuce
¼ cup fat-free Caesar dressing
⅓ cup shredded Parmesan cheese

1 To make croutons, preheat oven to 350°F. Place bread cubes in gallon-size resealable bag. Drizzle with oil and ½ teaspoon seasoning. Seal bag; shake until bread is evenly coated with oil and seasoning. Spread bread cubes in single layer on baking sheet. Bake 12 to 15 minutes, turning 2 or 3 times during baking, until bread is just crisp (bread will continue to crisp as it cools). Remove from oven; set aside.

2 Prepare grill for direct cooking. Season chicken with remaining seasoning. Grill chicken over medium heat, covered, about 8 to 10 minutes, turning once, until chicken is no longer pink in center. Remove from grill. Let stand 5 minutes.

3 Meanwhile, in large bowl, toss lettuce, dressing, cheese and croutons. Divide among four dinner plates. Cut chicken into strips and top each salad with chicken.

Makes 4 servings

nutrients per serving

Calories 270	**Total Fat** 12g	**Sodium** 564mg
Protein 20g	**Saturated Fat** 3g	**Fiber** 3g
Carbohydrate 22g	**Cholesterol** 42mg	

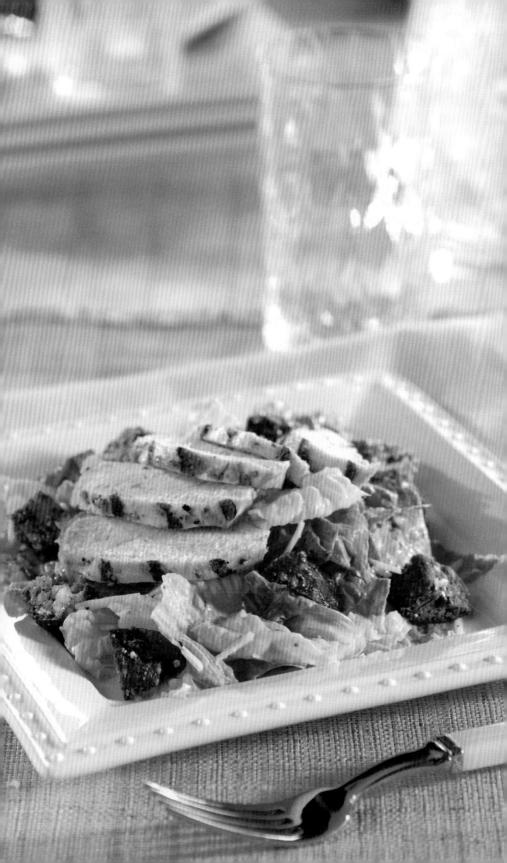

PIZZA, PASTA AND FLATBREADS

Tortilla Pizza Wedges

1 cup frozen corn, thawed
1 cup thinly sliced mushrooms
4 (6-inch) corn tortillas
¼ cup reduced-sodium pasta sauce
1 to 2 teaspoons chopped jalapeño pepper*
¼ teaspoon dried oregano
¼ teaspoon dried marjoram
½ cup (2 ounces) shredded part-skim mozzarella cheese

Jalapeño peppers can sting and irritate the skin, so wear rubber gloves when handling peppers and do not touch your eyes.

1 Preheat oven to 450°F. Spray large skillet with nonstick cooking spray; heat over medium heat. Add corn and mushrooms; cook and stir 4 to 5 minutes or until tender.

2 Place tortillas on baking sheet. Bake 4 minutes or until edges begin to brown.

3 Combine pasta sauce, jalapeño pepper, oregano and marjoram in small bowl. Spread evenly over tortillas. Top evenly with corn and mushrooms. Sprinkle with cheese.

4 Bake 4 to 5 minutes or until cheese is melted and pizzas are heated through. Cut each pizza into four wedges.

Makes 4 servings

nutrients per serving

Calories 155   **Total Fat** 4g   **Sodium** 136mg
Protein 7g   **Saturated Fat** 2g   **Fiber** 3g
Carbohydrate 24g   **Cholesterol** 8mg

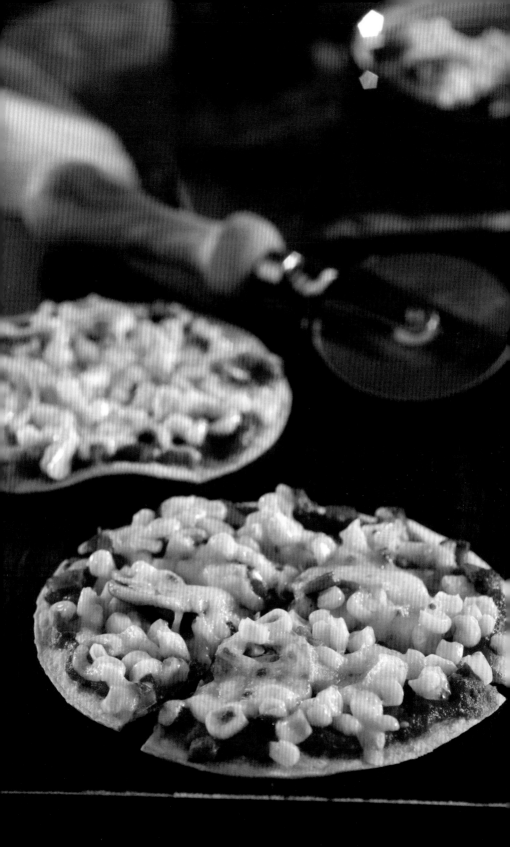

Chicken and Pasta Salad with Kalamata Olives

4 ounces uncooked multigrain rotini pasta
2 cups diced cooked chicken
½ cup chopped roasted red bell peppers
12 pitted kalamata olives, halved
1½ tablespoons olive oil
1 tablespoon dried basil
1 tablespoon cider vinegar
1 to 2 cloves garlic, minced
¼ teaspoon salt (optional)

1 Cook pasta according to package directions, omitting salt. Drain well; cool.

2 Combine chicken, peppers, olives, oil, basil, vinegar, garlic and salt, if desired, in large bowl.

3 Add cooled pasta to chicken mixture; toss gently. Divide equally among four plates.

Makes 4 servings

nutrients per serving

Calories 276	**Total Fat** 9g	**Sodium** 341mg
Protein 25g	**Saturated Fat** 2g	**Fiber** 3g
Carbohydrate 25g	**Cholesterol** 54mg	

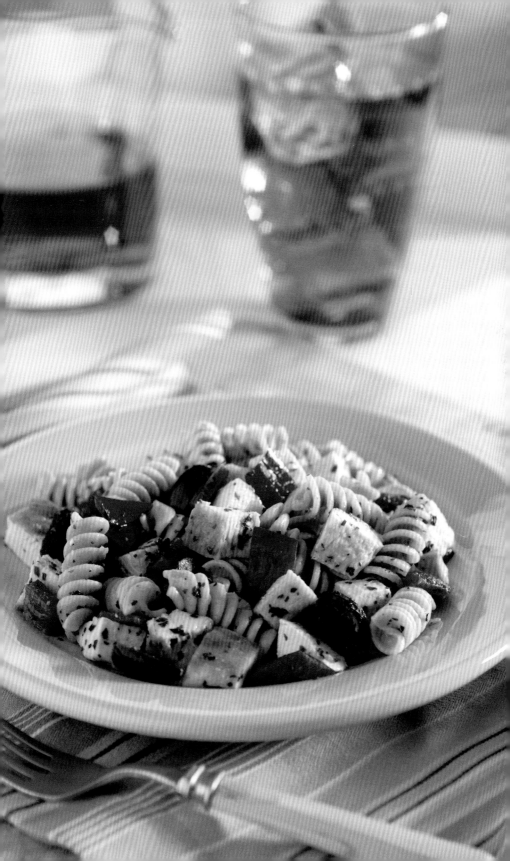

Summer's Bounty Pasta with Broccoli Pesto

2 cups broccoli florets
2 cups uncooked farfalle (bowtie pasta)
½ cup loosely packed fresh basil
5 tablespoons shredded Parmesan-Romano cheese, divided
2 tablespoons chopped walnuts, toasted*
1½ tablespoons extra virgin olive oil
2 cloves garlic, crushed and divided
⅛ teaspoon salt
6 ounces medium cooked shrimp
¼ teaspoon black pepper
1 package (6 ounces) fresh baby spinach
1 cup halved grape tomatoes

*To toast walnuts, spread in single layer in heavy skillet. Cook over medium heat 1 to 2 minutes or until nuts are lightly browned, stirring frequently.

1 Bring large saucepan of water to a boil. Add broccoli; cook 3 minutes or until tender. Remove to small bowl using slotted spoon; reserve water.

2 Cook pasta according to package directions using reserved water, omitting salt. Drain. Cover to keep warm.

3 Combine broccoli, basil, 3 tablespoons cheese, walnuts, oil, 1 clove garlic and salt in food processor or blender; process until smooth. Stir into pasta in saucepan; toss to coat. Cover to keep warm.

4 Spray large skillet with nonstick cooking spray; heat over medium heat. Add shrimp, remaining 1 clove garlic and pepper; cook until heated through. Stir in spinach and tomatoes; cook until spinach is wilted and tomatoes begin to soften. Stir into pasta.

5 Divide pasta mixture evenly among four serving bowls. Top with remaining 2 tablespoons cheese.

Makes 4 servings

nutrients per serving

Calories 263	**Total Fat** 12g	**Sodium** 638mg
Protein 20g	**Saturated Fat** 3g	**Fiber** 4g
Carbohydrate 22g	**Cholesterol** 94mg	

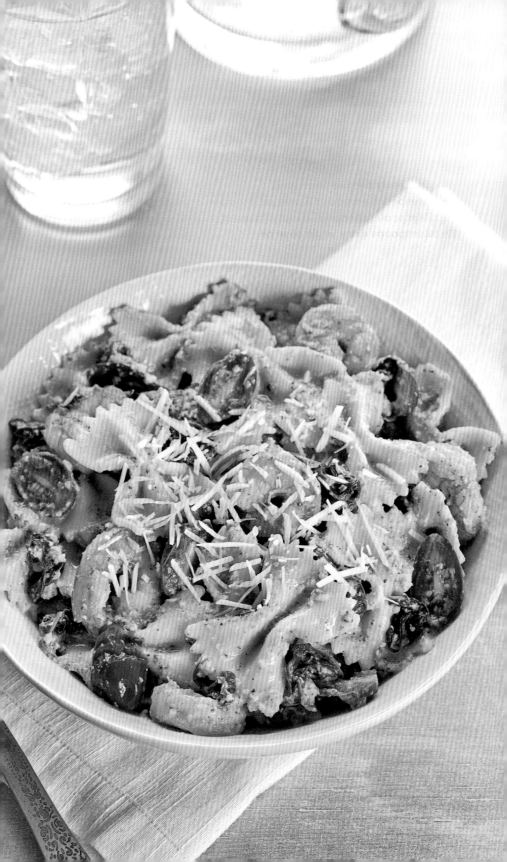

Grilled Steak and Blue Cheese Flatbreads

1 (4-ounce) filet mignon
¼ teaspoon garlic powder
⅛ teaspoon salt
⅛ teaspoon black pepper
2 light blue cheese spreadable cheese wedges (about 1 ounce each)
2 light original flatbreads
½ cup thinly sliced tomato
¼ cup thinly sliced red onion
2 tablespoons crumbled reduced-fat blue cheese
½ cup baby arugula
Balsamic vinegar (optional)

1 Prepare grill for direct cooking over medium heat.

2 Season filet with garlic powder, salt and pepper. Grill 5 minutes per side or until medium-rare or desired doneness. Remove to plate. Let stand 5 minutes. Reduce heat to low.

3 Slice filet into thin slices. Spread 1 cheese wedge onto each flatbread. Top evenly with filet slices, tomato and onion. Sprinkle with blue cheese.

4 Grill, covered, 8 to 10 minutes or until crisp and heated through. Top with arugula just before serving. Drizzle with balsamic vinegar, if desired.

Makes 4 appetizer or 2 main-dish servings (1 flatbread half per serving)

nutrients per serving

Calories 127
Protein 13g
Carbohydrate 10g

Total Fat 5g
Saturated Fat 2g
Cholesterol 19mg

Sodium 357mg
Fiber 5g

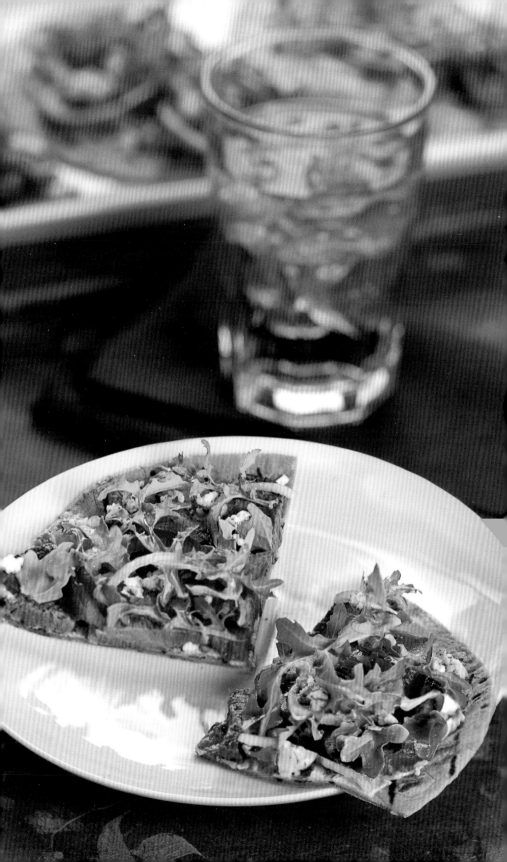

Onion and Shrimp Flatbread Pizza with Goat Cheese

4 teaspoons olive oil, divided
3 large onions, thinly sliced
¼ teaspoon salt
1 package (about 14 ounces) refrigerated pizza crust dough
½ pound small shrimp, peeled and deveined
⅛ cup chopped fresh chives
3 ounces goat cheese, crumbled
½ teaspoon black pepper (optional)

1 Heat 2 teaspoons oil in large skillet over medium heat. Add onions; cook and stir about 8 minutes. Stir in salt. Reduce heat to medium-low; cook, stirring occasionally, 25 minutes or until onions are soft and caramelized. If onions are cooking too fast, reduce heat to low.

2 Meanwhile, preheat oven to 425°F. Roll out dough on 15×10-inch baking sheet. Bake 8 to 10 minutes or until golden brown. Turn off oven. Spread caramelized onions over crust.

3 Heat remaining 2 teaspoons oil in same skillet over medium heat. Cook and stir shrimp 2 minutes or until pink and opaque. Arrange shrimp over onions on pizza. Sprinkle with chives, goat cheese and pepper, if desired.

4 Place pizza in warm oven 1 to 2 minutes or until cheese is soft. Cut into 12 squares.

Makes 6 servings (2 pieces per serving)

nutrients per serving

Calories 281
Protein 14g
Carbohydrate 38g

Total Fat 8g
Saturated Fat 3g
Cholesterol 63mg

Sodium 677mg
Fiber 2g

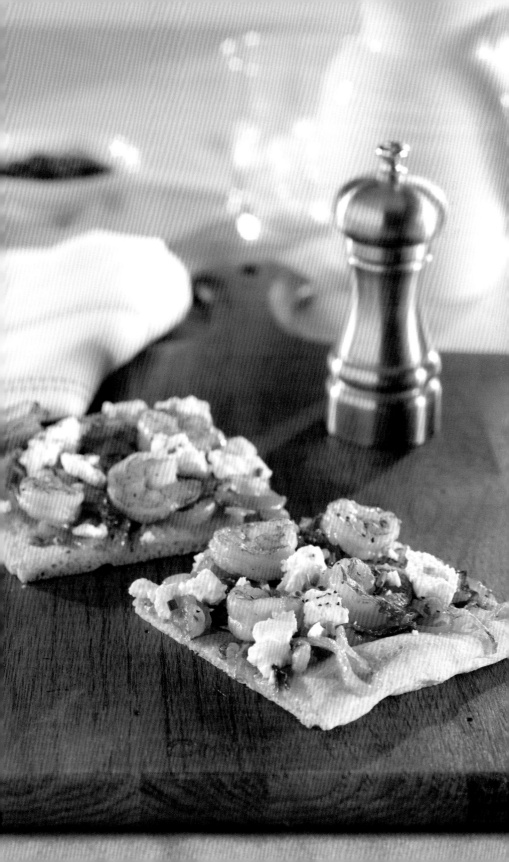

Herbed Chicken and Pasta with Spanish Olives

4 ounces uncooked rotini pasta

12 ounces boneless skinless chicken breasts, cut into bite-size pieces

½ teaspoon dried rosemary

¼ teaspoon dried thyme

¼ teaspoon red pepper flakes

4 cloves garlic, minced

1 cup grape tomatoes, quartered

3 ounces Spanish stuffed olives, halved lengthwise (about ½ cup)

2 tablespoons chopped fresh parsley

1½ cups packed baby spinach (1½ ounces), coarsely chopped

2 tablespoons extra virgin olive oil

⅛ teaspoon salt

1 Cook pasta according to package directions; drain and return to saucepan.

2 Meanwhile, spray large skillet with nonstick cooking spray and heat over medium-high heat. Cook and stir chicken, rosemary, thyme and pepper flakes 2 minutes or until chicken is slightly pink in center. Add garlic; cook and stir 15 seconds. Stir in tomatoes, olives and parsley; cook until heated through.

3 Add chicken mixture, spinach, oil and salt to pasta; toss until spinach begins to wilt.

Makes 4 servings (1 cup per serving)

nutrients per serving

Calories 254
Protein 21g
Carbohydrate 26g

Total Fat 11g
Saturated Fat 1g
Cholesterol 54mg

Sodium 538mg
Fiber 2g

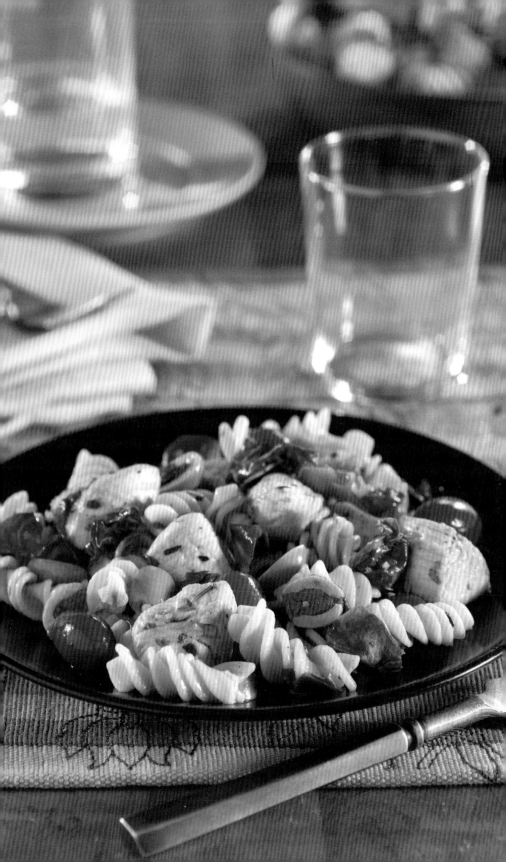

Mexican Pizza

1 package (about 14 ounces) refrigerated pizza crust dough
1 cup chunky salsa
1 teaspoon ground cumin
1 cup no-salt-added canned black beans, rinsed and drained*
1 cup frozen corn, thawed
½ cup sliced green onions
1½ cups shredded 2% Mexican cheese blend
½ cup chopped fresh cilantro (optional)

*Save the remaining ¾ cup beans (from a 15- or 16-ounce can) in the refrigerator for up to 4 days to add to salads or soups.

1 Preheat oven to 425°F. Unroll pizza dough onto 15×10×1-inch jelly-roll pan coated with nonstick cooking spray; press dough evenly to all edges of pan. Bake 8 minutes.

2 Combine salsa and cumin in small bowl; spread over partially baked crust. Top with beans, corn and onions. Bake 8 minutes or until crust is deep golden brown. Top with cheese; continue baking 2 minutes or until cheese is melted. Cut into squares; garnish with cilantro, if desired.

Makes 8 servings

nutrients per serving

Calories 241
Protein 23g
Carbohydrate 36g

Total Fat 6g
Saturated Fat 3g
Cholesterol 11mg

Sodium 699mg
Fiber 3g

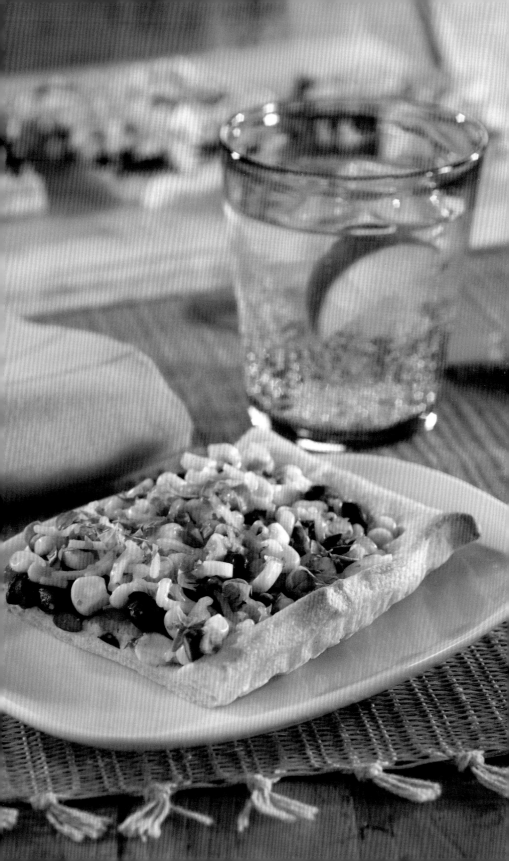

Pizza-Stuffed Potatoes

4 medium potatoes (about 7 ounces each)
¾ cup pizza sauce
⅛ teaspoon garlic powder
2 teaspoons grated Parmesan cheese
1 ounce turkey pepperoni slices (about 16), quartered
¾ cup shredded part-skim mozzarella cheese

1 Poke potatoes with fork and heat in microwave on HIGH 5 to 7 minutes or until soft. Split potatoes open with a knife; mash insides lightly.

2 Top each potato with 3 tablespoons pizza sauce and mix lightly into potato.

3 Sprinkle potatoes evenly with garlic powder and Parmesan cheese. Top evenly with pepperoni and mozzarella cheese.

4 Return potatoes to microwave and cook on HIGH 1 minute or until cheese is melted.

Makes 4 servings (1 potato per serving)

nutrients per serving

Calories 258
Protein 13g
Carbohydrate 42g

Total Fat 5g
Saturated Fat 2g
Cholesterol 23mg

Sodium 547mg
Fiber 5g

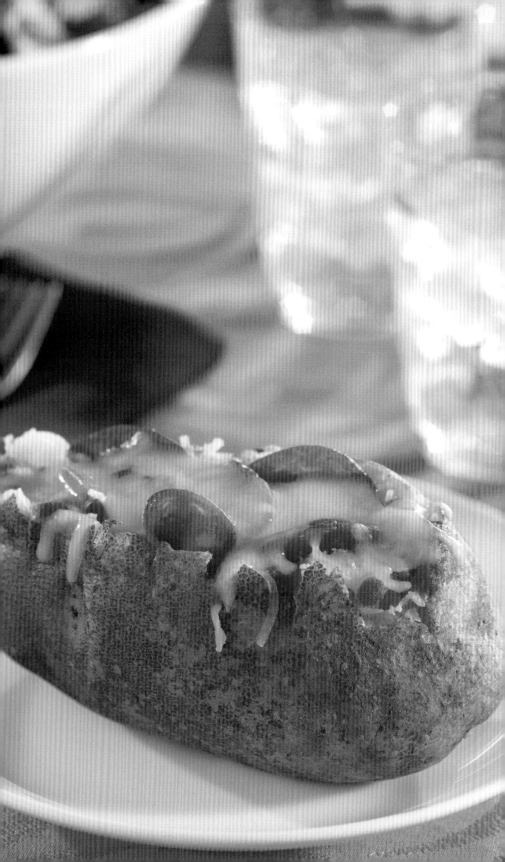

Grilled Pizza with Spinach and Artichokes

2 cloves garlic, finely minced
3 cups fresh spinach leaves, coarsely chopped
1 package (10 ounces) prepared whole wheat thin pizza crust
½ cup pizza sauce
1 cup chopped cooked chicken breast
½ cup chopped canned artichoke hearts, rinsed and drained
¾ cup shredded reduced-fat mozzarella cheese

1 Prepare grill for indirect cooking over medium heat.

2 Meanwhile, coat 8-inch skillet with nonstick cooking spray. Cook and stir garlic over medium heat 30 seconds. Stir in spinach. Cook and stir spinach and garlic until spinach is wilted. Remove from heat and drain spinach.

3 Place pizza crust on baking sheet. Spread sauce to within ½ inch of edge. Top with spinach mixture, chicken, artichokes and cheese. Transfer pizza to grill (do not put pan on grill). Grill over medium heat 3 to 5 minutes or until cheese is melted.

Makes 6 servings

nutrients per serving

Calories 238
Protein 16g
Carbohydrate 28g

Total Fat 7g
Saturated Fat 3g
Cholesterol 24mg

Sodium 460mg
Fiber 6g

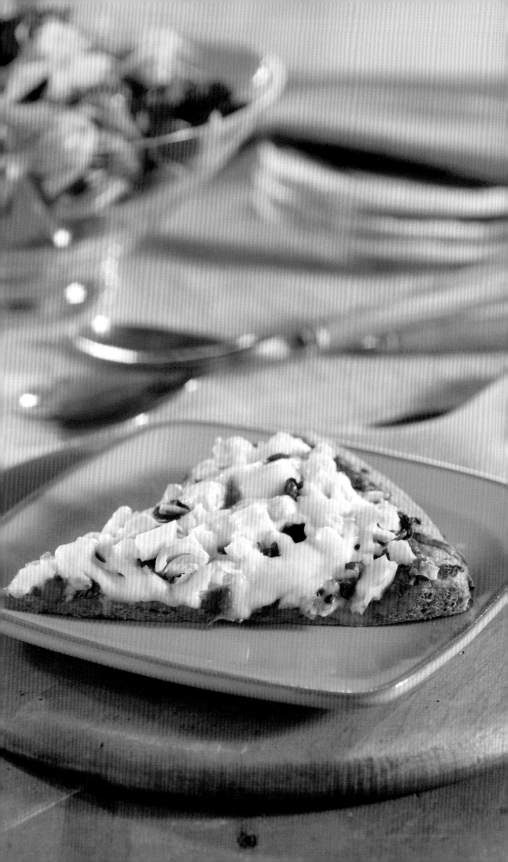

Broccoli and Shrimp Fettuccine

2 cups bite-size broccoli florets
4 ounces uncooked whole wheat fettuccine, broken in half
8 ounces medium shrimp, cooked
1⅓ cups fat-free (skim) milk, divided
1 tablespoon all-purpose flour
¼ teaspoon salt (optional)
⅛ teaspoon ground nutmeg
⅛ teaspoon black pepper
6 tablespoons grated Parmesan cheese, divided
16 grape tomatoes, halved
¼ cup chopped fresh Italian parsley

1 Steam broccoli 3 minutes or until tender. Bring large saucepan of water to a boil over high heat. Cook fettuccine according to package directions, omitting fat or salt. Add shrimp during last minute of cooking. Drain; keep warm in large serving bowl.

2 Meanwhile, whisk ⅔ cup milk, flour, salt, if desired, nutmeg and pepper in medium saucepan until smooth. Whisk in remaining ⅔ cup milk. Cook and stir over medium heat until mixture comes to a boil. Stir in 4 tablespoons cheese. Reduce heat to low; cook and stir 2 minutes.

3 Add broccoli, tomatoes, cheese sauce, remaining 2 tablespoons cheese and parsley to pasta and shrimp; mix well.

Makes 4 servings (1¼ cups per serving)

nutrients per serving

Calories 253	**Total Fat** 4g	**Sodium** 706mg
Protein 25g	**Saturated Fat** 2g	**Fiber** 4g
Carbohydrate 28g	**Cholesterol** 127mg	

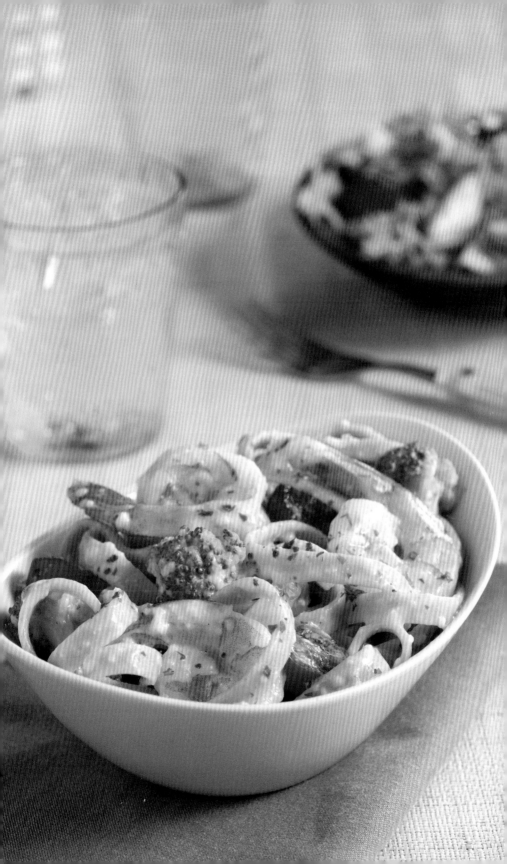

Veggie Pizza Pitas

2 whole wheat pita bread rounds, cut in half horizontally (to make 4 rounds)
¼ cup pizza sauce
1 teaspoon dried basil
⅛ teaspoon red pepper flakes (optional)
1 cup sliced mushrooms
½ cup thinly sliced green bell pepper
½ cup thinly sliced red onion
1 cup (4 ounces) shredded mozzarella cheese
2 teaspoons grated Parmesan cheese

1 Preheat oven to 475°F.

2 Arrange pita rounds, rough sides up, in single layer on large nonstick baking sheet. Spread 1 tablespoon pizza sauce evenly over each round to within ¼ inch of edge. Sprinkle with basil and pepper flakes, if desired. Top with mushrooms, bell pepper and onion. Sprinkle with mozzarella cheese.

3 Bake 5 minutes or until mozzarella cheese is melted. Sprinkle ½ teaspoon Parmesan cheese over each round.

Makes 4 servings (1 pizza per serving)

Note

These pizzas can be served as appetizers as well.

nutrients per serving

Calories 113	**Total Fat** 2g	**Sodium** 402mg
Protein 11g	**Saturated Fat** 1g	**Fiber** 2g
Carbohydrate 13g	**Cholesterol** 6mg	

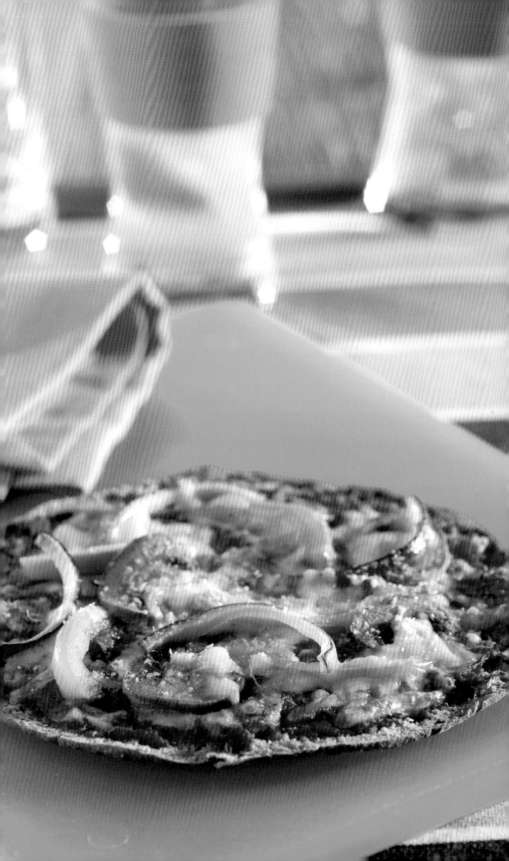

Artichoke and Tomato Pasta

8 ounces uncooked whole wheat spaghetti
1 can (14 ounces) artichoke hearts marinated in olive oil
1 medium onion, chopped
1 clove garlic, minced
¼ cup fat-free reduced-sodium vegetable *or* chicken broth
½ teaspoon Italian seasoning
1 pint cherry tomatoes, halved
3 tablespoons chopped fresh basil or parsley
¼ teaspoon salt
Black pepper (optional)
½ cup grated Parmesan cheese

1 Cook pasta according to package directions, omitting salt and fat; drain and return to saucepan.

2 Meanwhile, drain artichokes, reserving 1 tablespoon marinade; quarter artichokes and blot dry with paper towels. Set aside.

3 Heat reserved 1 tablespoon artichoke marinade in large skillet over medium-high heat. Add onion and garlic; cook and stir 3 minutes or until softened. Add broth and Italian seasoning; bring to a boil. Stir in artichokes and tomatoes; cook, covered, stirring occasionally, 6 to 8 minutes or until hot. Stir in basil, salt and pepper, if desired.

4 Add onion mixture to pasta; toss until blended. Sprinkle with cheese and serve immediately.

Makes 5 servings (1½ cups per serving)

nutrients per serving

Calories 269
Protein 13g
Carbohydrate 45g

Total Fat 6g
Saturated Fat 2g
Cholesterol 7mg

Sodium 385mg
Fiber 6g

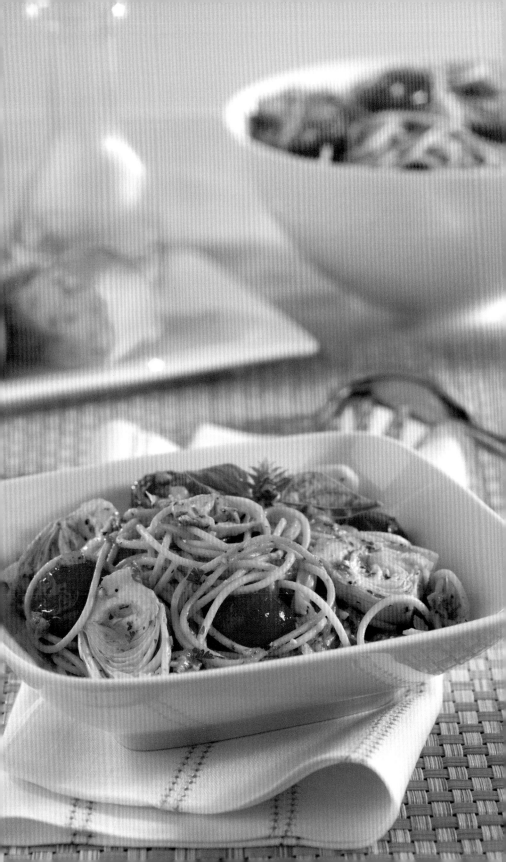

CHICKEN AND TURKEY

Tuscan Turkey and White Bean Skillet

1 teaspoon dried rosemary, divided
½ teaspoon garlic salt
½ teaspoon black pepper, divided
1 pound turkey breast cutlets, pounded to ¼-inch thickness
2 teaspoons canola oil, divided
1 can (about 15 ounces) no-salt-added navy beans *or* Great Northern beans, rinsed and drained
1 can (about 14 ounces) fire-roasted diced tomatoes
¼ cup grated Parmesan cheese

1 Combine ½ teaspoon rosemary, garlic salt and ¼ teaspoon pepper in small bowl; mix well. Sprinkle over turkey.

2 Heat 1 teaspoon oil in large nonstick skillet over medium heat. Add half of turkey; cook 2 to 3 minutes per side or until no longer pink in center. Remove to platter; tent with foil to keep warm. Repeat with remaining 1 teaspoon oil and turkey.

3 Add beans, tomatoes, remaining ½ teaspoon rosemary and ¼ teaspoon pepper to skillet; bring to a boil over high heat. Reduce heat to low; simmer 5 minutes.

4 Spoon bean mixture over turkey; sprinkle with cheese.

Makes 6 servings (1 cup per serving)

nutrients per serving

Calories 230	**Total Fat** 4g	**Sodium** 334mg
Protein 25g	**Saturated Fat** 1g	**Fiber** 9g
Carbohydrate 23g	**Cholesterol** 36mg	

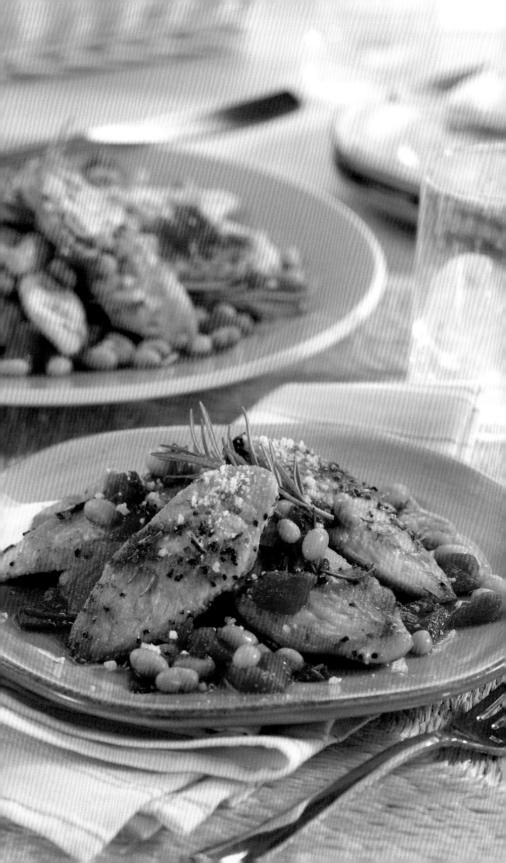

Turkey Sliders

1 pound extra lean ground turkey
¼ cup finely chopped green onions
2 tablespoons low-fat mayonnaise
1 tablespoon Worcestershire sauce
¼ teaspoon black pepper
⅛ teaspoon salt
12 baby spinach leaves
¼ cup (1 ounce) shredded reduced-fat sharp Cheddar cheese
1 shallot, thinly cut into 12 slices
1 tablespoon steak sauce (optional)
12 mini whole wheat pita bread rounds, cut in half horizontally

1 Combine turkey, onions, mayonnaise, Worcestershire sauce, pepper and salt in large bowl; mix well. Shape into 12 patties.

2 Spray large nonstick skillet with nonstick cooking spray; heat over medium heat. Add patties; cook 5 minutes per side or until cooked through.

3 Layer spinach, patties, cheese, shallot and steak sauce, if desired, evenly on pita bottoms. Cover with pita tops.

Makes 6 servings (2 sliders per serving)

Note

There are different varieties of ground turkey available. Regular ground turkey (85% lean) is a combination of white and dark meat, which is comparable in fat to some lean cuts of ground beef. Ground turkey breast is lowest in fat (up to 99% lean), but it can dry out very easily when grilled. To keep the best texture, gently form patties or meatballs and do not press down on the patties as they grill.

nutrients per serving

Calories 262 **Total Fat** 4g **Sodium** 596mg
Protein 24g **Saturated Fat** 1g **Fiber** 2g
Carbohydrate 31g **Cholesterol** 43mg

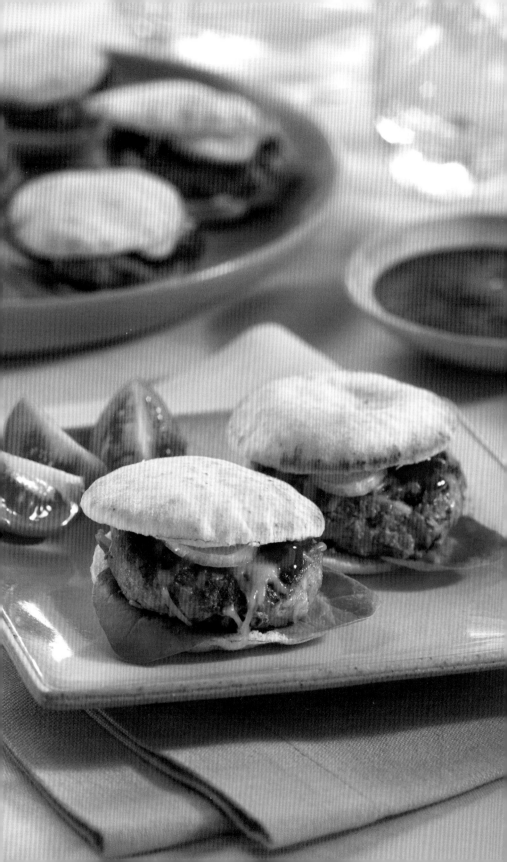

Mushroom & Chicken Skillet

1 pound boneless skinless chicken breasts, cut into bite-size pieces
1 can (about 14 ounces) fat-free chicken broth
½ teaspoon dried thyme
2 cups uncooked instant rice
8 ounces mushrooms, thinly sliced
1 can (10¾ ounces) 98% fat-free cream of celery soup
Chopped fresh parsley

1 Cook chicken in broth and ¼ cup hot water in 12-inch nonstick skillet until mixture comes to a full boil. Stir in thyme and rice, making sure rice is covered with broth. Place mushrooms on top (the steam will cook the thin slices of mushrooms). Cover skillet; turn off heat and let stand 5 minutes.

2 Turn heat to low; cook 2 minutes, gently stirring soup and mushrooms into chicken and rice. Continue stirring until ingredients are combined and hot. Sprinkle with parsley before serving.

Makes 4 servings (1½ cups per serving)

Tip

Serve with mixed greens salad and sliced fresh strawberries.

nutrients per serving

Calories 277	**Total Fat** 4g	**Sodium** 774mg
Protein 32g	**Saturated Fat** 1g	**Fiber** 2g
Carbohydrate 28g	**Cholesterol** 67mg	

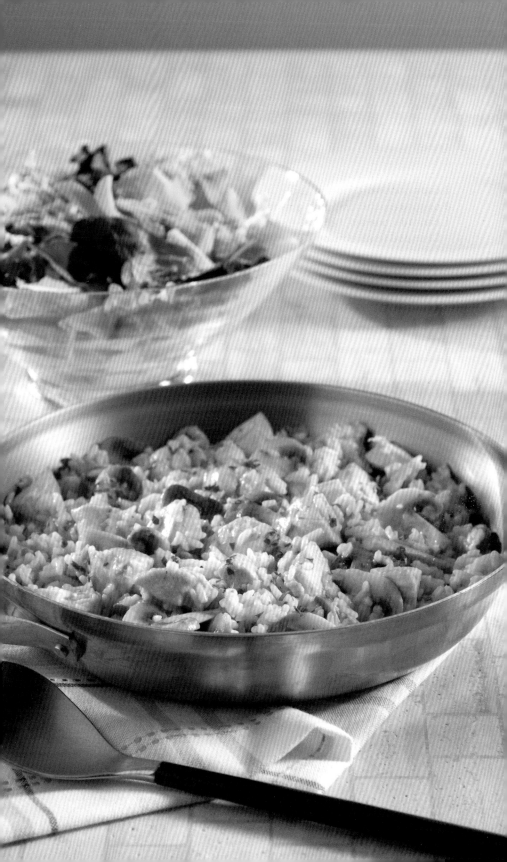

Tuscan Pasta

1 pound boneless skinless chicken breasts, cut into 1-inch pieces
2 cans (about 14 ounces each) Italian-style stewed tomatoes, undrained
1 can (about 15 ounces) red kidney beans, rinsed and drained
1 can (15 ounces) tomato sauce
1 cup water
1 jar (4½ ounces) sliced mushrooms, drained
1 medium green bell pepper, chopped
½ cup chopped onion
½ cup chopped celery
4 cloves garlic, minced
1 teaspoon Italian seasoning
6 ounces uncooked thin spaghetti, broken in half

Slow Cooker Directions

1 Place all ingredients except spaghetti in slow cooker.

2 Cover; cook on LOW 4 hours or until vegetables are tender.

3 Stir in spaghetti. Turn slow cooker to HIGH. Cook 10 minutes; stir. Cover; cook 35 minutes or until pasta is tender.

Makes 8 servings

nutrients per serving

Calories 266	**Total Fat** 2g	**Sodium** 814mg
Protein 21g	**Saturated Fat** 1g	**Fiber** 6g
Carbohydrate 40g	**Cholesterol** 34mg	

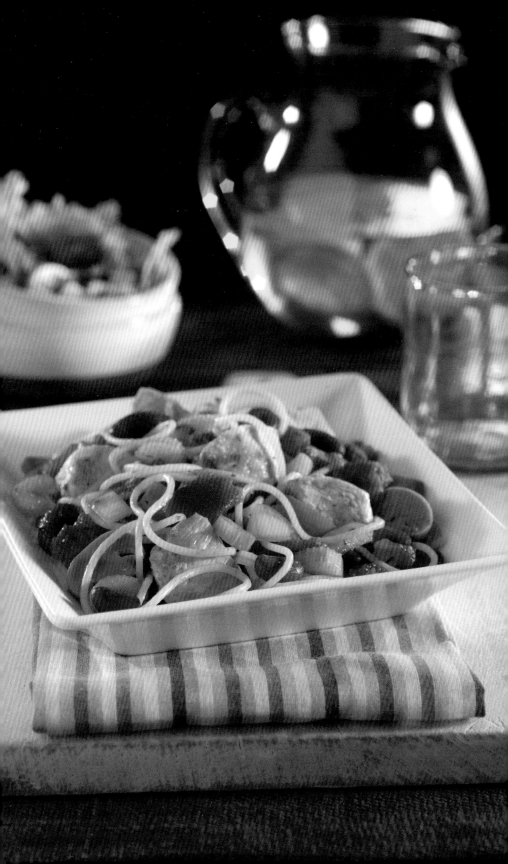

Turkey Piccata

3 tablespoons all-purpose flour
¼ teaspoon salt
¼ teaspoon black pepper
2 egg whites
1 teaspoon water
⅔ cup plain dry bread crumbs
1 package (about 17½ ounces) turkey breast cutlets or slices
3 teaspoons butter, divided
3 teaspoons olive oil, divided
2 cloves garlic, minced
¾ to 1 cup fat-free reduced-sodium chicken broth
2 tablespoons capers, rinsed and drained
2 tablespoons lemon juice
2 tablespoons chopped fresh parsley
1 teaspoon grated lemon peel

1 Combine flour, salt and pepper in small resealable food storage bag. Beat egg white and water in small shallow bowl. Place bread crumbs on small shallow plate. Add 1 cutlet to bag; shake to coat lightly with flour mixture. Dip cutlet in egg mixture; let excess drip off. Roll in bread crumbs; press each side to coat. Repeat with remaining cutlets. Discard any remaining flour, egg and crumb mixture.

2 Heat 1 teaspoon butter and 1 teaspoon oil in large nonstick skillet over medium heat. Add half of cutlets; cook about 3 minutes on each side or until golden brown and no longer pink in center. Remove to plate and keep warm. Repeat with 1 teaspoon butter, 1 teaspoon oil and remaining cutlets.

3 Heat remaining 1 teaspoon butter and 1 teaspoon oil in same skillet. Add garlic; cook 1 minute. Stir in broth, capers and lemon juice; simmer 1 to 2 minutes or until sauce is slightly reduced. Pour sauce over cutlets; sprinkle with parsley and lemon peel.

Makes 4 servings (2 cutlets per serving)

nutrients per serving

Calories 296	**Total Fat** 9g	**Sodium** 551mg
Protein 34g	**Saturated Fat** 3g	**Fiber** 1g
Carbohydrate 19g	**Cholesterol** 59mg	

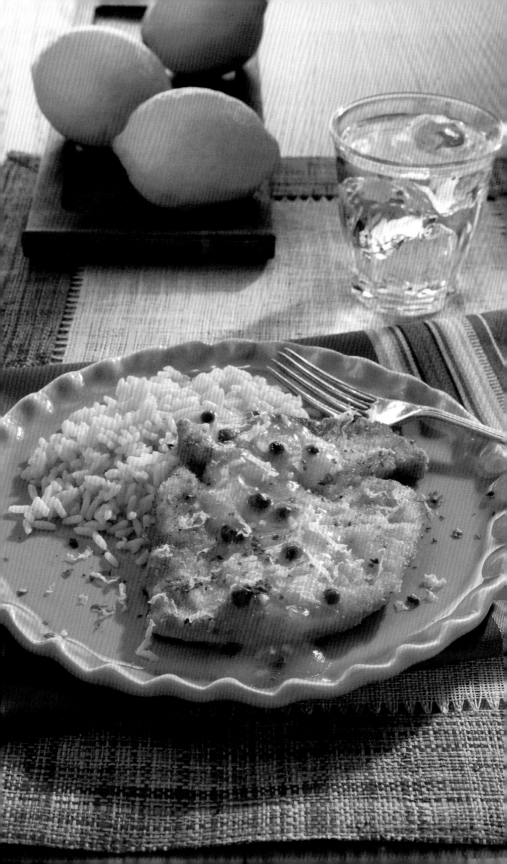

Crispy Baked Chicken

8 ounces (1 cup) fat-free French onion dip
½ cup fat-free (skim) milk
1 cup cornflake crumbs
½ cup wheat germ
6 skinless chicken breasts or thighs (about 1½ pounds)

1 Preheat oven to 350°F. Spray shallow baking pan with nonstick cooking spray.

2 Place dip in shallow bowl; stir until smooth. Add milk, 1 tablespoon at a time, until pourable consistency is reached.

3 Combine cornflake crumbs and wheat germ on plate.

4 Dip chicken pieces in milk mixture, then roll in cornflake mixture. Place chicken in single layer in prepared pan. Bake 45 to 50 minutes or until juices run clear when chicken is pierced with fork and chicken is no longer pink in center.

Makes 6 servings (1 breast per serving)

nutrients per serving

Calories 253	**Total Fat** 2g	**Sodium** 437mg
Protein 35g	**Saturated Fat** 1g	**Fiber** 1g
Carbohydrate 22g	**Cholesterol** 66mg	

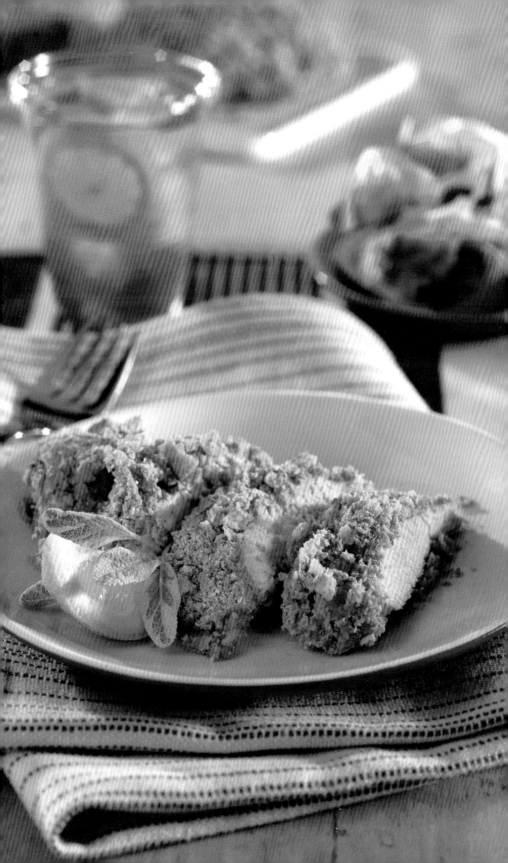

Turkey & Veggie Roll-Ups

2 tablespoons hummus, any flavor
1 (8-inch) whole wheat tortilla
¼ cup sliced baby spinach
2 slices oven-roasted turkey breast (about 1 ounce)
¼ cup thinly sliced English cucumber
1 slice (1 ounce) reduced-fat Swiss cheese
¼ cup thinly sliced carrot

Spread hummus on tortilla to within 1 inch of edge. Layer with spinach, turkey, cucumber, cheese and carrots. Roll up tortilla and filling; cut into four pieces.

Makes 2 servings (2 roll-ups per serving)

nutrients per serving

Calories 140	**Total Fat** 4g	**Sodium** 292mg
Protein 11g	**Saturated Fat** 1g	**Fiber** 2g
Carbohydrate 14g	**Cholesterol** 16mg	

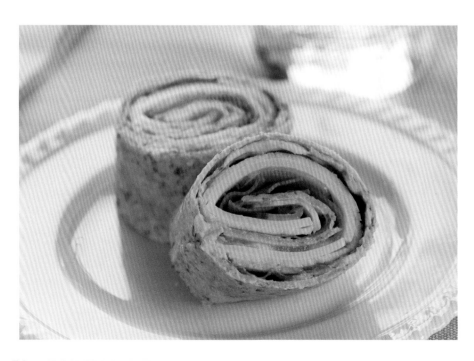

Slow Cooker Turkey Breast

1 turkey breast (about 3 pounds)
Garlic powder
Paprika
Dried parsley flakes

Slow Cooker Directions

1 Place turkey in slow cooker. Season with garlic powder, paprika and parsley. Cover; cook on LOW 6 to 8 hours or until internal temperature reaches 170°F.

2 Remove turkey to cutting board; cover with foil and let stand 10 to 15 minutes before carving. (Internal temperature will rise 5° to 10°F during stand time.)

Makes 4 to 6 servings (4 ounces per serving)

nutrients per serving

Calories 140
Protein 27g
Carbohydrate 0g

Total Fat 3g
Saturated Fat 1g
Cholesterol 79mg

Sodium 41mg
Fiber 0g

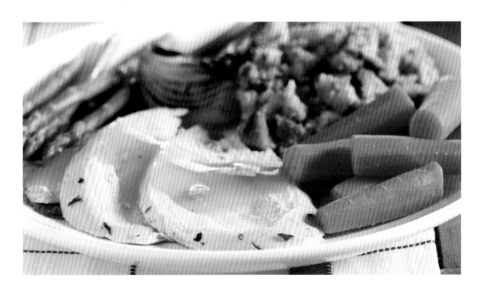

Kale & Mushroom Stuffed Chicken Breasts

3 teaspoons olive oil, divided
1 cup coarsely chopped mushrooms
2 cups thinly sliced kale
1 tablespoon fresh lemon juice
½ teaspoon salt, divided
4 boneless skinless chicken breasts (about 4 ounces each)
¼ cup crumbled fat-free feta cheese
¼ teaspoon black pepper

1 Heat 1 teaspoon oil in large skillet over medium-high heat. Add mushrooms; cook and stir 5 minutes or until mushrooms begin to brown. Add kale; cook and stir 8 minutes or until wilted. Sprinkle with lemon juice and ¼ teaspoon salt. Remove to small bowl. Let stand 5 to 10 minutes to cool slightly.

2 Meanwhile, place each chicken breast between plastic wrap. Pound with meat mallet or rolling pin to about ½-inch thickness.

3 Gently stir feta cheese into mushroom and kale mixture. Spoon ¼ cup mixture down center of each chicken breast. Roll up to enclose filling; secure with toothpicks. Sprinkle with remaining ¼ teaspoon salt and pepper.

4 Wipe out same skillet with paper towels. Heat remaining 2 teaspoons oil in skillet over medium heat. Add chicken; brown on all sides. Cover and cook 5 minutes per side or until no longer pink. Remove toothpicks before serving.

Makes 4 servings (1 breast per serving)

Serving Suggestion

Serve this flavorful entrée with a fresh salad or summer vegetables.

nutrients per serving

Calories 192	**Total Fat** 7g	**Sodium** 495mg
Protein 29g	**Saturated Fat** 1g	**Fiber** 1g
Carbohydrate 4g	**Cholesterol** 73mg	

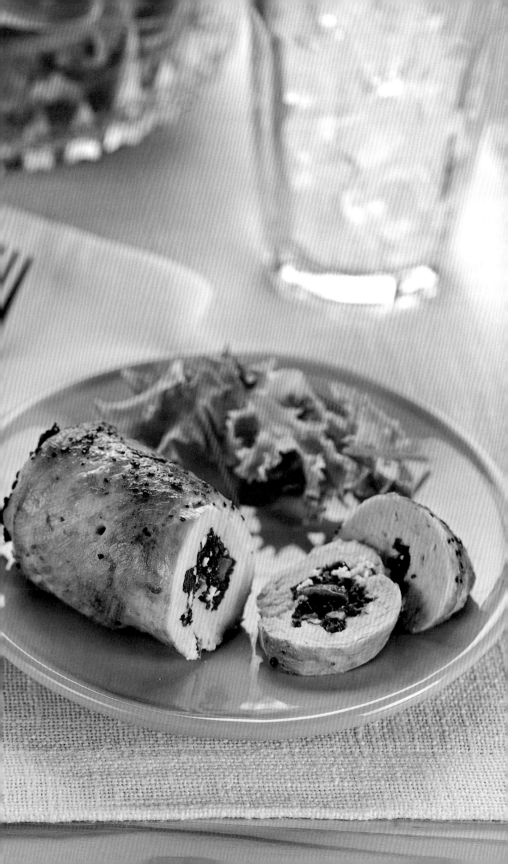

Chicken Mirabella

4 boneless skinless chicken breasts (about 4 ounces each)
½ cup pitted prunes
½ cup assorted pitted olives (black, green and/or a combination)
¼ cup light white grape juice *or* **white wine**
2 tablespoons olive oil
1 tablespoon capers
1 tablespoon red wine vinegar
1 teaspoon dried oregano
1 clove garlic, minced
½ teaspoon chopped fresh parsley, plus additional for garnish
2 teaspoons packed brown sugar

1 Preheat oven to 350°F.

2 Place chicken in 8-inch baking dish. Combine prunes, olives, grape juice, oil, capers, vinegar, oregano, garlic and ½ teaspoon parsley in medium bowl. Pour evenly over chicken. Sprinkle with brown sugar.

3 Bake 25 to 30 minutes or until no longer pink in center, basting with sauce halfway through. Garnish with additional parsley.

Makes 4 servings

Serving Suggestion

Serve with long-grain and wild rice which offers protein, fiber, and many minerals, including iron, and some vitamins.

Tip

For more intense flavor, marinate chicken at least 8 hours or overnight and sprinkle with brown sugar just before baking.

nutrients per serving

Calories 280	**Total Fat** 11g	**Sodium** 113mg
Protein 25g	**Saturated Fat** 2g	**Fiber** 2g
Carbohydrate 20g	**Cholesterol** 72mg	

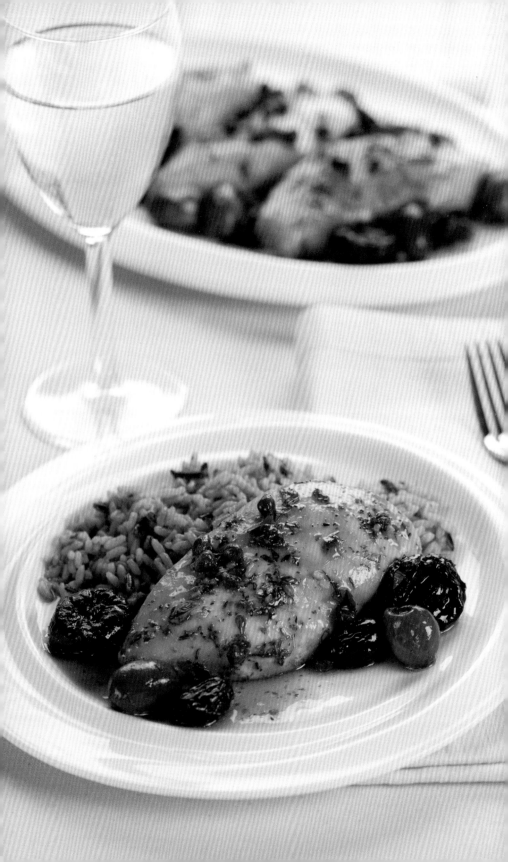

Turkey Sausage & Spinach Stuffed Shells

18 uncooked jumbo shell pasta
1 teaspoon olive oil
8 ounces spicy Italian turkey sausage, casings removed
½ cup chopped onion
2 cloves garlic, minced
1 package (6 ounces) baby spinach
1 cup fat-free ricotta cheese
1½ cups tomato-basil pasta sauce, divided
½ cup shredded Parmesan cheese, divided
¼ chopped fresh basil

1 Preheat oven to 375°F. Cook pasta according to package directions; drain.

2 Meanwhile, heat oil in large nonstick skillet over medium heat. Add sausage, onion and garlic; cook 5 minutes or until sausage begins to brown, stirring to break up meat. Add spinach in batches; cook and stir until wilted. Remove from heat; stir in ricotta cheese, ½ cup pasta sauce and ¼ cup Parmesan cheese.

3 Arrange shells in 2-quart casserole. Fill shells evenly with turkey mixture. Spoon remaining 1 cup pasta sauce evenly over shells. Cover with foil.

4 Bake 30 to 35 minutes or until heated through. Top with remaining ¼ cup Parmesan cheese and basil.

Makes 6 servings (3 filled shells per serving)

nutrients per serving

Calories 255	**Total Fat** 5g	**Sodium** 580mg
Protein 15g	**Saturated Fat** 2g	**Fiber** 4g
Carbohydrate 36g	**Cholesterol** 24mg	

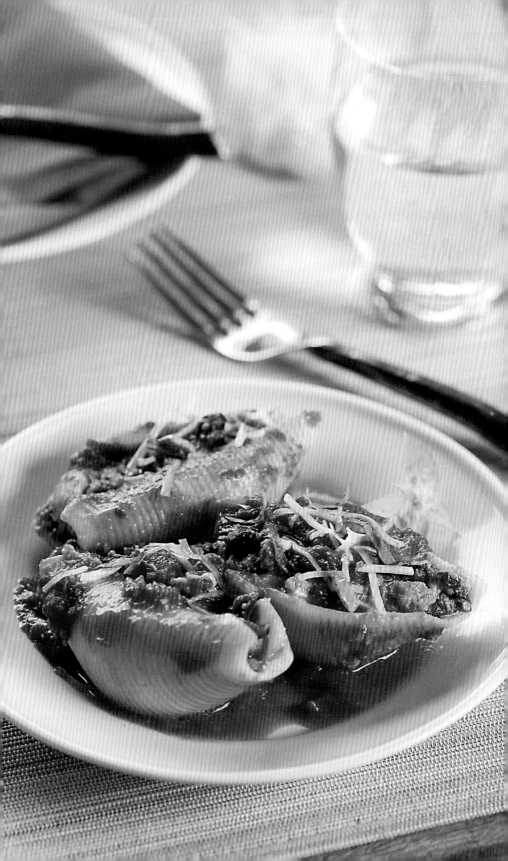

Mu Shu Turkey

1 can (16 ounces) plums, drained and pitted
½ cup orange juice
¼ cup finely chopped onion
1 tablespoon minced fresh ginger
¼ teaspoon ground cinnamon
1 pound boneless turkey breast, cut into thin strips
6 (7-inch) flour tortillas
3 cups coleslaw mix

Slow Cooker Directions

1 Place plums in blender or food processor. Cover; process until almost smooth. Combine plums, orange juice, onion, ginger and cinnamon in slow cooker; mix well.

2 Place turkey over plum mixture. Cover; cook on LOW 3 to 4 hours.

3 Remove turkey from slow cooker. Divide evenly among tortillas. Spoon about 2 tablespoons plum sauce over turkey in each tortilla; top each with about ½ cup coleslaw mix. Fold bottom edge of tortilla over filling; fold in sides. Roll up to completely enclose filling. Use remaining plum sauce for dipping.

Makes 6 servings (1 filled tortilla per serving)

nutrients per serving

Calories 248
Protein 17g
Carbohydrate 36g

Total Fat 4g
Saturated Fat 1g
Cholesterol 30mg

Sodium 282mg
Fiber 3g

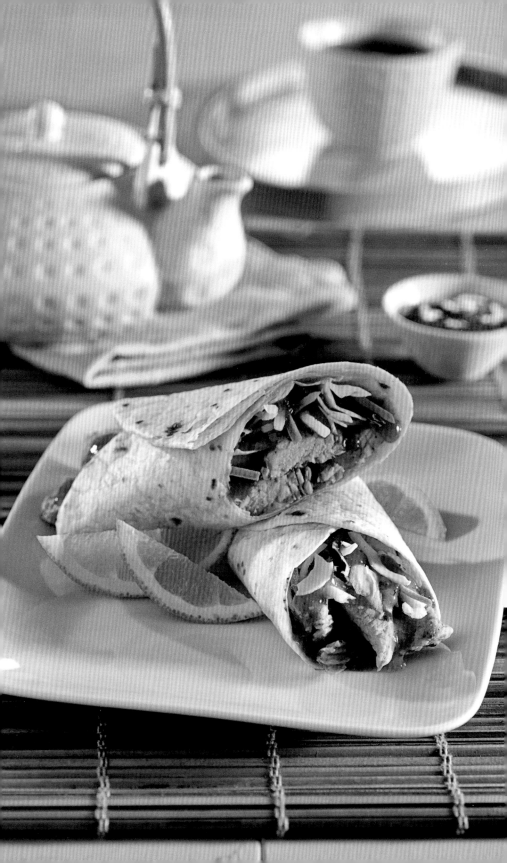

BEEF AND PORK

Authentic Meat Loaf

¾ cup no-salt-added tomato sauce, divided
2 egg whites
4 tablespoons reduced-sodium chunky salsa, divided
½ teaspoon black pepper
½ cup 100% whole grain oats (oatmeal)
½ cup finely minced onion
⅓ cup canned no-salt-added mushroom stems and pieces, drained and
   chopped
1 clove garlic, finely minced
8 ounces lean ground turkey
8 ounces 96% lean ground beef

1 Preheat oven to 350°F. Spray foil with nonstick cooking spray. Place foil on broiler pan; set aside.

2 Mix ½ cup tomato sauce, egg whites, 3 tablespoons salsa and pepper in medium bowl. Stir in oatmeal, onion, mushrooms and garlic.

3 Place ground turkey and ground beef in large bowl; mix lightly to combine. Stir in tomato mixture; mix well.

4 Transfer meat mixture to prepared pan; shape into 4×8-inch rectangular loaf. Mix remaining ¼ cup tomato sauce and 1 tablespoon salsa in small bowl; drizzle on top of meat loaf.

5 Bake 55 minutes or until cooked through (165°F). Let stand 5 minutes before slicing.

Makes 4 servings

nutrients per serving

Calories 220	**Total Fat** 7g	**Sodium** 300mg
Protein 26g	**Saturated Fat** 2g	**Fiber** 3g
Carbohydrate 13g	**Cholesterol** 60mg	

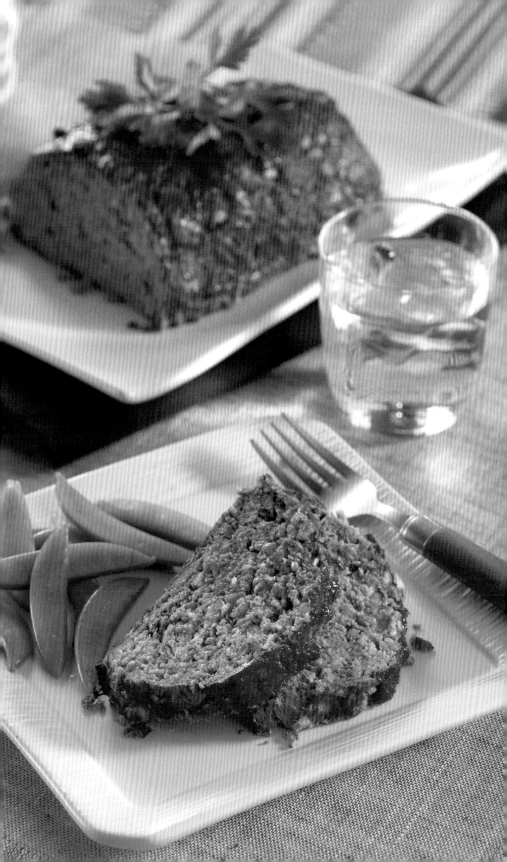

Beef and Pineapple Kabobs

1 boneless beef top sirloin or top round steak (about 1 pound)
1 small onion, finely chopped
½ cup teriyaki sauce
16 pieces (1-inch cubes) fresh pineapple
1 can (8 ounces) water chestnuts, drained

1 Cut steak into ¼-inch-thick strips. For marinade, combine onion and teriyaki sauce in small bowl. Add beef strips, stirring to coat.

2 Alternately thread beef strips (weaving back and forth), pineapple cubes and water chestnuts onto bamboo or thin metal skewers. (If using bamboo skewers, soak in water for 20 to 30 minutes before using to prevent them from burning.)

3 Place kabobs on grid over medium coals. Grill 4 minutes, turning once, or until meat is cooked through. Serve immediately.

Makes 4 servings (1 kabob per serving)

Note
Recipe can also be prepared with flank steak.

Serving Suggestion
Serve with hot cooked rice and stir-fried broccoli, mushrooms and red bell peppers.

nutrients per serving

Calories 232	**Total Fat** 3g	**Sodium** 880mg
Protein 38g	**Saturated Fat** 3g	**Fiber** 1g
Carbohydrate 26g	**Cholesterol** 101mg	

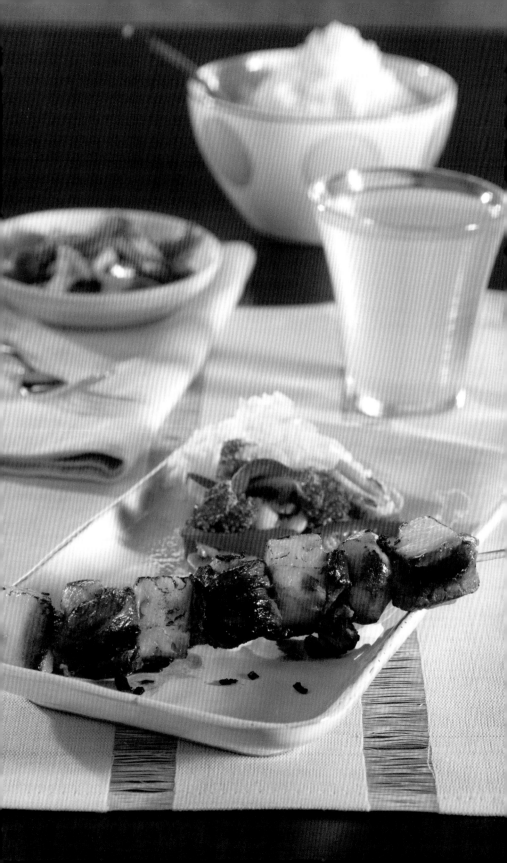

Garlic Pork with Roasted Red Potatoes

½ teaspoon paprika
½ teaspoon garlic powder
1 pound pork tenderloin
1 tablespoon extra virgin olive oil
6 new potatoes, scrubbed and quartered (12 ounces total)
1 teaspoon dried oregano
½ teaspoon salt
½ teaspoon black pepper

1 Preheat oven to 425°F. Coat 13×9-inch baking pan with nonstick cooking spray; set aside.

2 Combine paprika and garlic powder in small bowl; sprinkle evenly over pork.

3 Coat large skillet with nonstick cooking spray; heat over medium-high heat. Brown pork 3 minutes, turn and cook 3 minutes. Place in center of baking pan.

4 Remove skillet from heat. Add oil, potatoes and oregano; toss until well coated. Arrange potato mixture around pork, scraping sides and bottom of skillet with rubber spatula. Combine salt and pepper in small bowl; sprinkle evenly over all. Bake, uncovered, 22 minutes or until pork reaches 155°F to 160°F.

5 Remove pork to cutting board; let stand 5 minutes before slicing. Stir potatoes, cover with foil and let stand while pork is resting. Serve pork with potatoes.

Makes 4 servings (3 ounces cooked pork and about ½ cup potatoes per serving)

nutrients per serving

Calories 229	**Total Fat** 6g	**Sodium** 344mg
Protein 25g	**Saturated Fat** 1g	**Fiber** 2g
Carbohydrate 18g	**Cholesterol** 73mg	

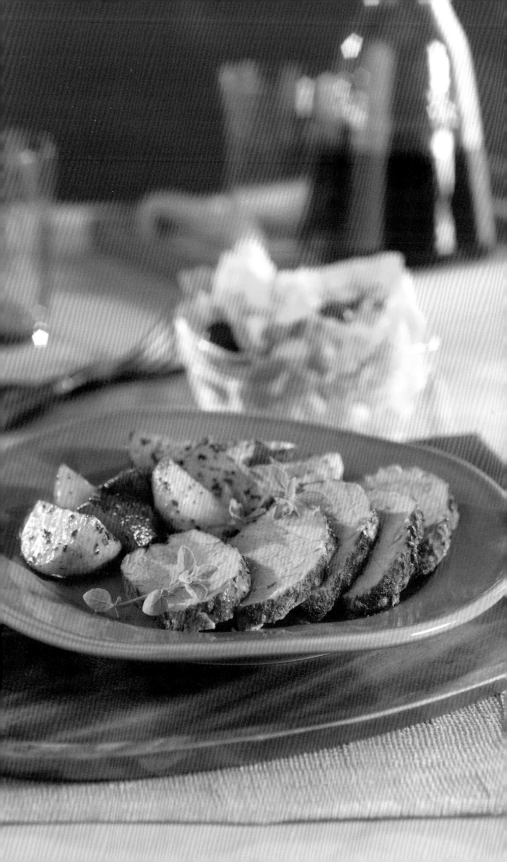

Texas-Style Barbecued Brisket

3 tablespoons Worcestershire sauce
2 cloves garlic, minced
1 tablespoon chili powder
1 teaspoon celery salt
1 teaspoon black pepper
1 teaspoon liquid smoke
1 beef brisket (3 to 4 pounds), trimmed
2 bay leaves
    Barbecue Sauce (recipe follows)

nutrients per serving

Calories 275	Saturated Fat 3g
Protein 24g	Cholesterol
Carbohydrate	73mg
20g	Sodium 658mg
Total Fat 11g	Fiber 1g

Slow Cooker Directions

1 Combine Worcestershire sauce, garlic, chili powder, celery salt, pepper and liquid smoke in small bowl. Spread mixture on all sides of beef. Place beef in large resealable food storage bag; seal bag. Refrigerate 24 hours.

2 Place beef, marinade and bay leaves in slow cooker, cutting meat in half to fit, if necessary. Cover; cook on LOW 7 hours. Meanwhile, prepare Barbecue Sauce.

3 Remove beef from slow cooker and pour juices into 2-cup measure; let stand 5 minutes. Skim fat from juices. Remove and discard bay leaves. Stir 1 cup juices into Barbecue Sauce. Discard remaining juices.

4 Return beef and sauce mixture to slow cooker. Cover; cook on LOW 1 hour or until meat is fork-tender. Remove beef to cutting board. Cut across grain into ¼-inch-thick slices. Serve with Barbecue Sauce.

Makes 10 to 12 servings

Barbecue Sauce

2 tablespoons vegetable oil
1 onion, chopped
2 cloves garlic, minced
1 cup ketchup
½ cup molasses
¼ cup cider vinegar
2 teaspoons chili powder
½ teaspoon dry mustard

nutrients per serving

Calories 40	Saturated Fat 0g
Protein 0g	Cholesterol 0mg
Carbohydrate 7g	Sodium 135mg
Total Fat 1g	Fiber 0g

1 Heat oil in medium saucepan over medium heat. Add onion and garlic; cook and stir until onion is tender.

2 Add remaining ingredients. Simmer over medium heat 5 minutes.

Makes about 1¾ cups

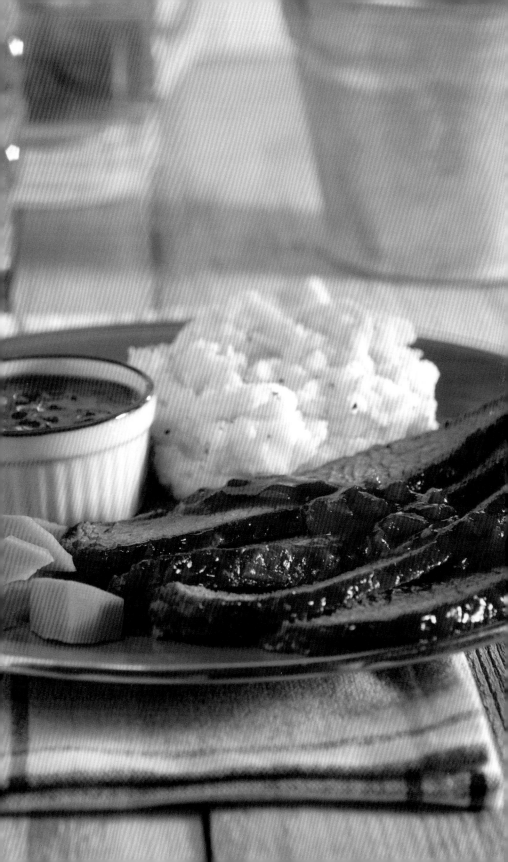

Apple-Cherry Glazed Pork Chops

¼ to ½ teaspoon dried thyme
⅛ teaspoon salt
⅛ teaspoon black pepper
2 boneless pork loin chops (3 ounces each), trimmed of fat
⅔ cup unsweetened apple juice
½ small apple, sliced
2 tablespoons sliced green onion
2 tablespoons dried tart cherries
1 teaspoon cornstarch
1 tablespoon water

1 Combine thyme, salt and pepper in small bowl. Rub onto both sides of pork chops.

2 Spray large skillet with nonstick cooking spray; heat over medium heat. Add pork chops; cook 3 to 5 minutes or until barely pink in center, turning once. Remove to plate; keep warm.

3 Add apple juice, apple slices, green onion and cherries to same skillet. Simmer 2 to 3 minutes or until apple and onion are tender.

4 Stir cornstarch into water in small bowl until smooth; stir into skillet. Bring to a boil; cook and stir until thickened. Spoon apple mixture over pork chops.

Makes 2 servings (1 pork chop with ½ cup apple glaze per serving)

nutrients per serving

Calories 243
Protein 19g
Carbohydrate 23g

Total Fat 8g
Saturated Fat 3g
Cholesterol 40mg

Sodium 191mg
Fiber 1g

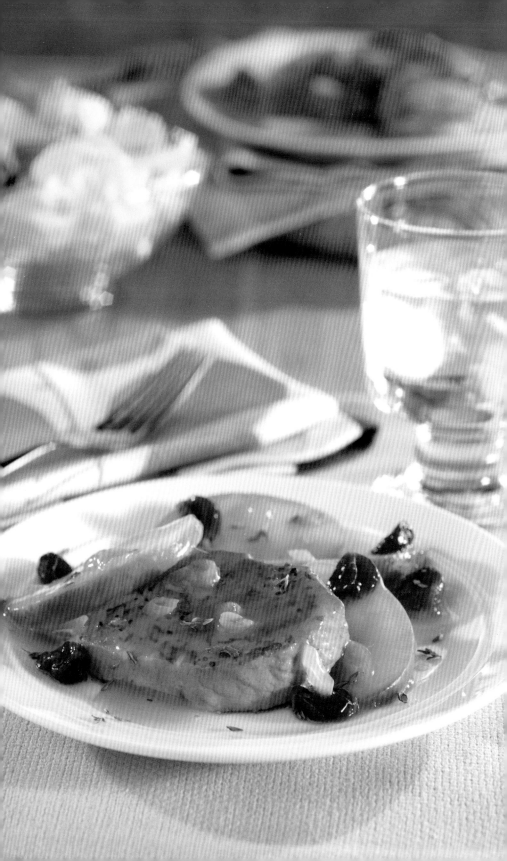

Red Wine & Oregano Beef Kabobs

¼ cup dry red wine
¼ cup finely chopped fresh parsley
2 tablespoons Worcestershire sauce
1 tablespoon reduced-sodium soy sauce
1 teaspoon dried oregano
3 cloves garlic, minced
½ teaspoon salt (optional)
½ teaspoon black pepper
¾ pound boneless beef top sirloin steak, cut into 16 (1-inch) pieces
16 whole mushrooms (about 8 ounces total)
1 medium red onion, cut in eighths and layers separated

1 Combine wine, parsley, Worcestershire sauce, soy sauce, oregano, garlic, salt, if desired, and pepper in small bowl; stir until well blended. Place steak, mushrooms and onion in large resealable food storage bag. Add wine mixture; toss. Seal and marinate in the refrigerator 1 hour, turning frequently.

2 Soak four (12-inch) or eight (6-inch) bamboo skewers in water for 20 minutes to prevent burning.

3 Preheat broiler. Alternate beef, mushrooms and two layers of onion on skewers.

4 Coat broiler rack with nonstick cooking spray. Arrange skewers on broiler rack; brush with marinade. Broil 4 to 6 inches from heat source 8 to 10 minutes, turning occasionally.

Makes 4 servings (one 12-inch kabob per serving)

Tip
Pair the kabob with a side of whole grain brown rice, if your diet permits.

nutrients per serving

Calories 163	**Total Fat** 4g	**Sodium** 209mg
Protein 22g	**Saturated Fat** 1g	**Fiber** 1g
Carbohydrate 8g	**Cholesterol** 40mg	

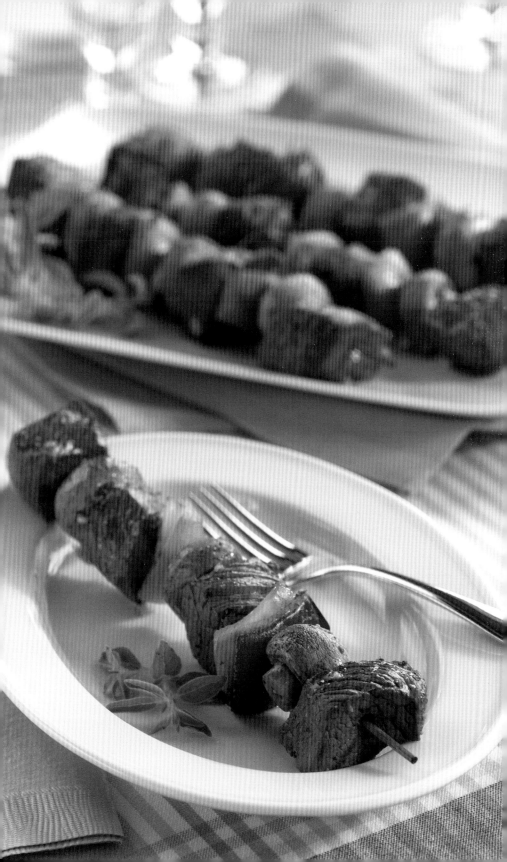

Garlic Beef

1 teaspoon sesame oil
1 pound beef eye of round, trimmed, cut into thin strips
1 package (10 ounces) frozen chopped broccoli
1 tablespoon minced garlic
1 tablespoon light soy sauce
¼ teaspoon black pepper

Heat oil in 12-inch nonstick skillet over high heat. Add beef, broccoli, garlic, soy sauce and pepper. Cook, stirring occasionally, 15 minutes or until beef is done.

Makes 4 servings (1 cup per serving)

nutrients per serving

Calories 214	**Total Fat** 9g	**Sodium** 320mg
Protein 27g	**Saturated Fat** 3g	**Fiber** 2g
Carbohydrate 6g	**Cholesterol** 42mg	

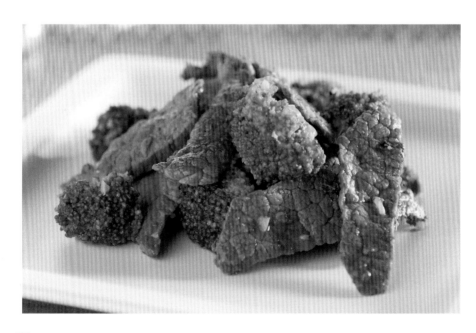

Maple & Sage Pork Chops

2 tablespoons finely chopped fresh sage, plus additional for garnish
2 teaspoons olive oil
½ teaspoon salt
4 boneless pork chops (about 4 ounces each)
2 teaspoons maple syrup

1 Combine 2 tablespoons sage, oil and salt in small bowl. Rub mixture evenly over pork chops. Place on rimmed baking sheet.

2 Broil pork chops 4 minutes. Turn over; brush evenly with syrup. Broil 4 minutes or until pork chops are browned and barely pink in center. Garnish with additional sage.

Makes 4 servings

Serving Suggestion

This delicious dish is perfect for a cold day. Serve it with fresh roasted vegetables to combine the unique flavors of fall with the delightful flavor of the tender pork.

nutrients per serving

Calories 203	**Total Fat** 10g	**Sodium** 342mg
Protein 25g	**Saturated Fat** 3g	**Fiber** 0g
Carbohydrate 2g	**Cholesterol** 62mg	

Mini Meatloaves

3 tablespoons ketchup
1 tablespoon balsamic vinegar
1 tablespoon olive oil
1½ cups finely chopped onion
1½ cups finely chopped mushrooms
1½ cups chopped baby spinach
1½ pounds extra lean ground sirloin
¾ cup old-fashioned oats
2 egg whites
½ teaspoon salt
½ teaspoon black pepper

1 Preheat oven to 375°F. Spray six mini (4¼×2½-inch) loaf pans with nonstick cooking spray. Whisk ketchup and vinegar in small bowl until smooth and well blended; set aside.

2 Heat oil in large skillet over medium heat. Add onion, mushrooms and spinach; cook and stir 8 minutes or until tender. Remove to large bowl. Let stand until cool enough to handle.

3 Add beef, oats, egg whites, salt and pepper to vegetables; mix well. Divide mixture evenly among prepared pans. Brush half of ketchup mixture evenly over loaves.

4 Bake 15 minutes. Brush with remaining ketchup mixture. Bake 5 minutes or until cooked through (160°F).

Makes 6 servings (1 mini meatloaf per serving)

nutrients per serving

Calories 270
Protein 28g
Carbohydrate 14g

Total Fat 11g
Saturated Fat 3g
Cholesterol 62mg

Sodium 362mg
Fiber 2g

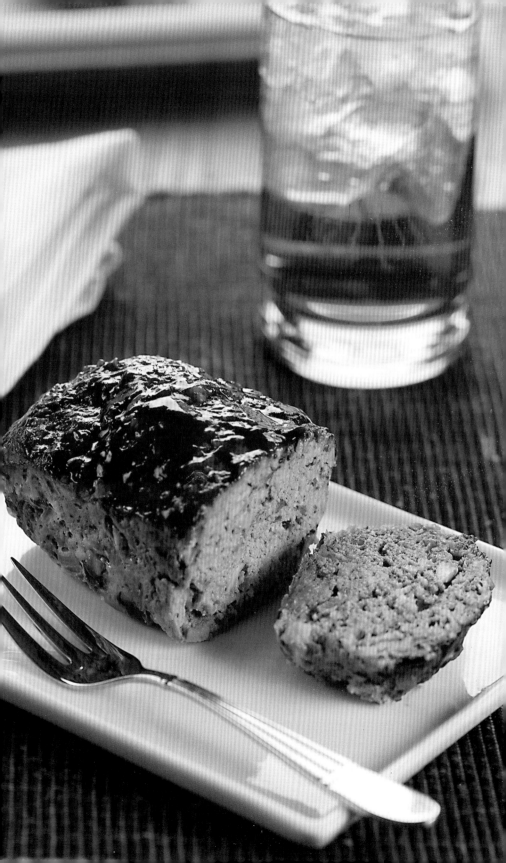

FISH AND SEAFOOD

Pasta and Tuna Filled Peppers

¾ cup uncooked ditalini pasta
4 large green bell peppers
1 cup chopped seeded fresh tomatoes
1 can (about 6 ounces) white tuna packed in water, drained and flaked
½ cup chopped celery
½ cup (2 ounces) shredded reduced-fat Cheddar cheese
¼ cup fat-free mayonnaise or salad dressing
1 teaspoon salt-free garlic and herb seasoning
2 tablespoons shredded reduced-fat Cheddar cheese (optional)

1 Cook pasta according to package directions, omitting salt. Rinse and drain; set aside.

2 Cut thin slice from top of each bell pepper; remove seeds and membranes from insides. Rinse bell peppers; place, cut side down, on paper towels to drain.*

3 Combine cooked pasta, tomatoes, tuna, celery, ½ cup cheese, mayonnaise and seasoning in large bowl until well blended; spoon evenly into bell pepper shells.

4 Place on large microwavable plate; cover with waxed paper. Microwave on HIGH 7 to 8 minutes, turning halfway through cooking time. Top evenly with 2 tablespoons cheese before serving, if desired.

For more tender bell peppers, cook in boiling water 2 minutes. Plunge into cold water, drain upside-down on paper towels before filling.

Makes 4 servings (1 stuffed pepper per serving)

nutrients per serving

Calories 216
Protein 19g
Carbohydrate 27g

Total Fat 4g
Saturated Fat 1g
Cholesterol 26mg

Sodium 574mg
Fiber 2g

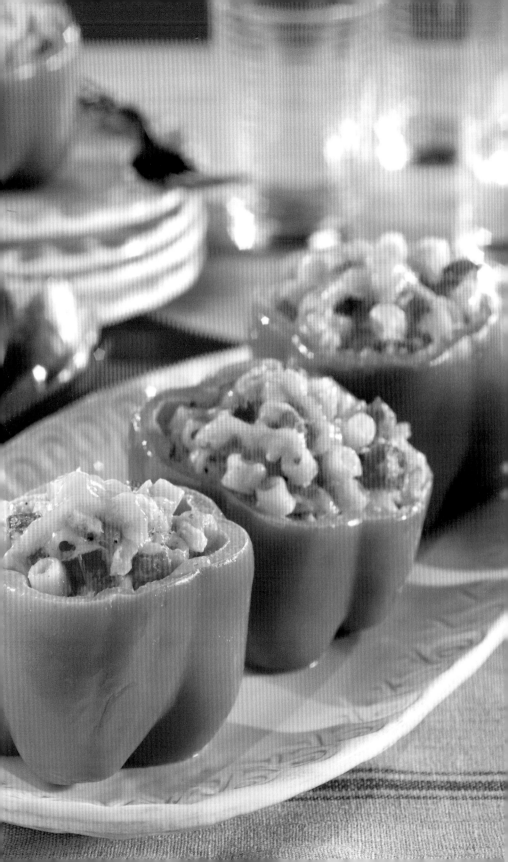

Oriental Baked Cod

2 tablespoons reduced-sodium soy sauce
2 tablespoons apple juice
1 tablespoon finely chopped fresh ginger
2 cloves garlic, minced
1 teaspoon crushed Szechuan peppercorns
4 cod fillets (about 1 pound)
4 green onions, thinly sliced

1 Preheat oven to 375°F. Spray roasting pan with nonstick cooking spray.

2 Whisk soy sauce, apple juice, ginger, garlic and peppercorns in small bowl until well blended. Place fish in prepared pan; pour soy sauce mixture over fish.

3 Bake 10 minutes or until fish is opaque and flakes easily when tested with fork.

4 Remove fish to serving dish; pour pan juices over fish. Sprinkle with green onions.

Makes 4 servings (1 fillet per serving)

nutrients per serving

Calories 100   **Total Fat** 1g   **Sodium** 329mg
Protein 20g   **Saturated Fat** 1g   **Fiber** 1g
Carbohydrate 3g   **Cholesterol** 45mg

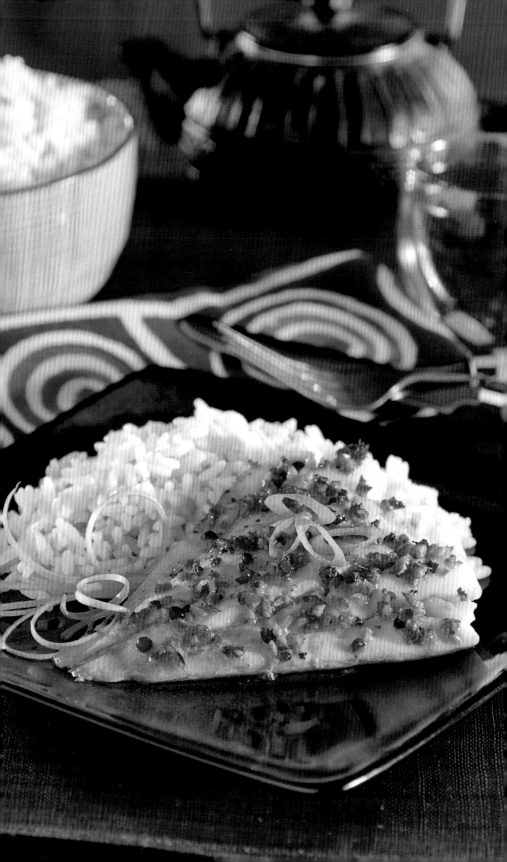

Garlic Skewered Shrimp

1 pound raw large shrimp, peeled and deveined
2 tablespoons reduced-sodium soy sauce
1 tablespoon vegetable oil
3 cloves garlic, minced
¼ teaspoon red pepper flakes (optional)
3 green onions, cut into 1-inch pieces

1 Prepare grill for direct cooking over medium heat. Soak four (12-inch) wooden skewers in hot water 30 minutes. Meanwhile, place shrimp in large resealable food storage bag. Combine soy sauce, oil, garlic and red pepper flakes, if desired, in cup; mix well. Pour over shrimp. Seal bag; turn to coat. Marinate at room temperature 15 minutes.

2 Drain shrimp; reserve marinade. Alternately thread shrimp and onions onto skewers. Brush with reserved marinade; discard any remaining marinade. Grill, covered, 5 minutes per side or until shrimp are pink and opaque.

Makes 4 servings (1 skewer per serving)

Serving Suggestion
For a more attractive presentation, leave the tails on the shrimp.

nutrients per serving

Calories 128	**Total Fat** 4g	**Sodium** 464mg
Protein 20g	**Saturated Fat** 1g	**Fiber** 1g
Carbohydrate 2g	**Cholesterol** 173mg	

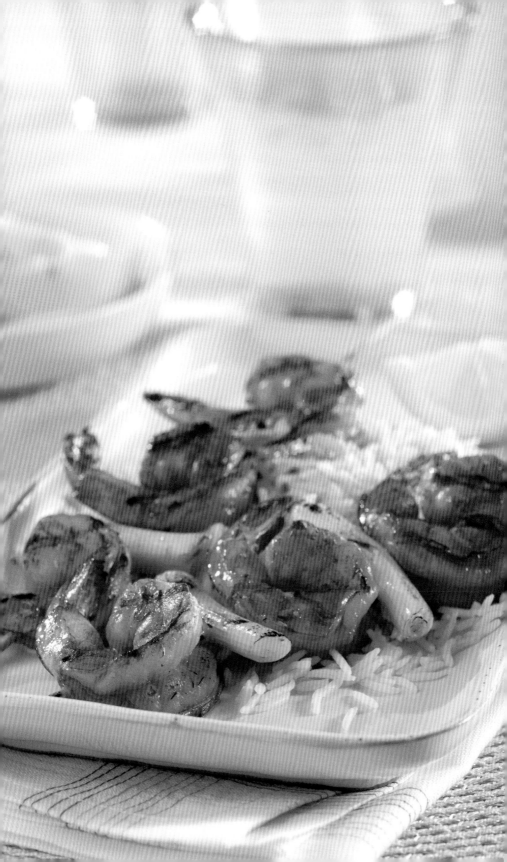

Deviled Crab Bake

2 teaspoons canola oil
½ cup diced onion
½ cup diced green bell pepper
¼ cup diced celery
1 cup fresh bread crumbs
¼ cup reduced-fat (2%) milk
1 can (about 6½ ounces) crabmeat, drained
1 teaspoon dried dill
1 tablespoon lemon juice
Pinch ground red pepper or seafood seasoning mix
Pinch black pepper

1 Preheat oven to 375°F.

2 Heat ovenproof skillet over medium heat. Add oil; heat. Add onion, bell pepper and celery. Cook, stirring frequently, 2 to 3 minutes or until onion is translucent and vegetables are tender-crisp. Remove from heat and set aside.

3 Place bread crumbs in mixing bowl. Dribble milk over crumbs to moisten, while stirring lightly. Let mixture stand 5 minutes.

4 Add crab, cooked vegetables, dill, lemon juice and red and black pepper. Stir lightly to blend. Spoon mixture back into ovenproof skillet. Bake 15 minutes or until lightly browned.

Makes 2 servings (1½ cups per serving)

nutrients per serving

Calories 230　　**Total Fat** 7g　　**Sodium** 480mg
Protein 23g　　**Saturated Fat** 1g　　**Fiber** 2g
Carbohydrate 19g　　**Cholesterol** 65mg

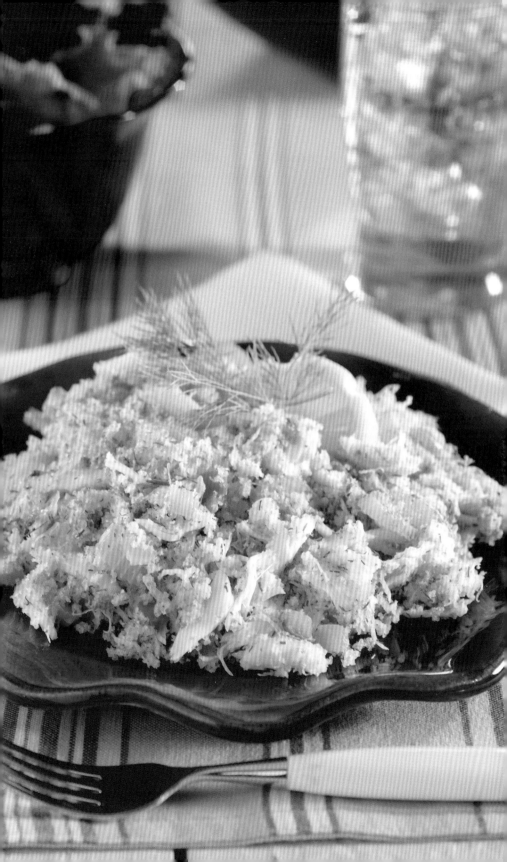

Crisp Lemony Baked Fish

1¼ cups crushed cornflakes
¼ cup grated Parmesan cheese
2 tablespoons minced green onions (green parts only)
⅛ teaspoon black pepper
1 lemon
¼ cup egg substitute
4 small haddock fillets (about 3 ounces each)

1 Preheat oven to 400°F. Line baking sheet with parchment paper.

2 Combine cornflakes, cheese, green onions and pepper on large plate. Grate lemon; stir peel into cornflake mixture. Reserve lemon.

3 Pour egg substitute into shallow bowl. Dip fish fillets into egg substitute, then into cornflake mixture; coat well on both sides. Place coated fillets on prepared baking sheet.

4 Bake 10 minutes or until fish begins to flake when tested with fork. Cut reserved lemon into wedges; serve with fish.

Makes 4 servings

nutrients per serving

Calories 209	**Total Fat** 2g	**Sodium** 364mg
Protein 22g	**Saturated Fat** 1g	**Fiber** 1g
Carbohydrate 26g	**Cholesterol** 53mg	

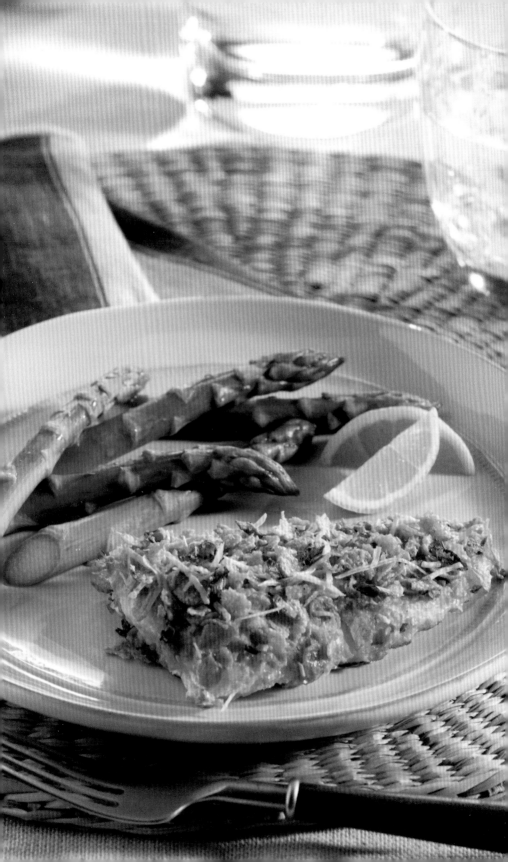

Fresh Garlic Shrimp Linguine

6 ounces uncooked multigrain linguine or spaghetti, broken in half
½ pound raw shrimp, peeled and deveined
¼ cup grated Parmesan cheese
3 tablespoons light margarine
1 clove garlic, minced
½ teaspoon seafood seasoning
¼ cup finely chopped fresh parsley (optional)
⅛ teaspoon salt (optional)

1 Cook linguine according to package directions, omitting salt and fat, about 7 minutes or until al dente. Add shrimp; cook 3 to 4 minutes or until shrimp are pink and opaque. Drain; transfer to medium bowl.

2 Add cheese, margarine, garlic and seafood seasoning; toss gently to coat. Add parsley and salt, if desired; toss to combine.

Makes 4 servings (1 cup per serving)

nutrients per serving

Calories 270　　**Total Fat** 7g　　**Sodium** 242mg
Protein 21g　　**Saturated Fat** 2g　　**Fiber** 3g
Carbohydrate 30g　　**Cholesterol** 91mg

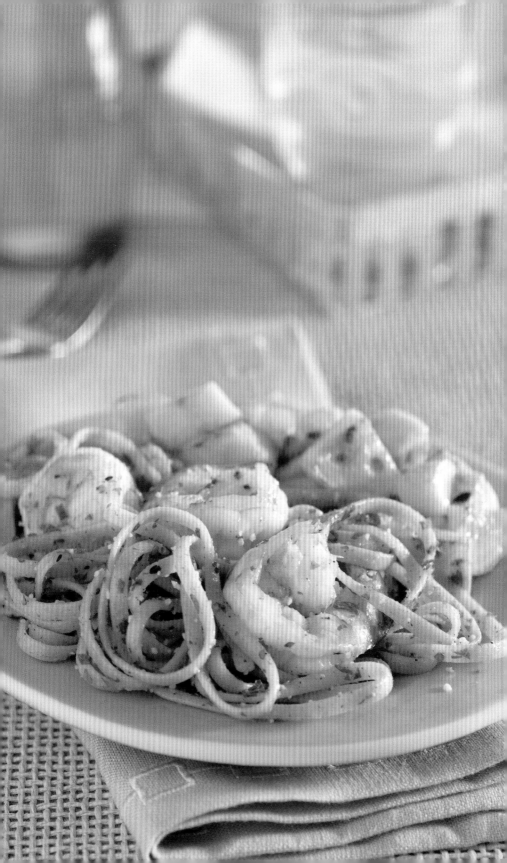

Grilled Salmon Fillets, Asparagus and Onions

½ teaspoon paprika
6 salmon fillets (6 to 8 ounces *each*)
⅓ cup bottled honey-Dijon marinade or barbecue sauce
1 bunch (about 1 pound) fresh asparagus spears, ends trimmed
1 large red or sweet onion, cut into ¼-inch slices
1 tablespoon olive oil
Salt and black pepper

1 Prepare grill for direct grilling. Sprinkle paprika over salmon fillets. Brush marinade over salmon; let stand at room temperature 15 minutes.

2 Brush asparagus and onion slices with oil; season to taste with salt and pepper.

3 Place salmon, skin side down, in center of grill grid. Place asparagus and onion slices around salmon. Grill, covered, 5 minutes. Turn salmon and vegetables. Grill 5 to 6 minutes more or until salmon flakes when tested with fork and vegetables are crisp-tender. Separate onion slices into rings; serve over asparagus.

Makes 6 servings (1 salmon fillet and ¾ cup asparagus/onion mixture per serving)

nutrients per serving

Calories 255
Protein 35g
Carbohydrate 8g

Total Fat 8g
Saturated Fat 1g
Cholesterol 86mg

Sodium 483mg
Fiber 2g

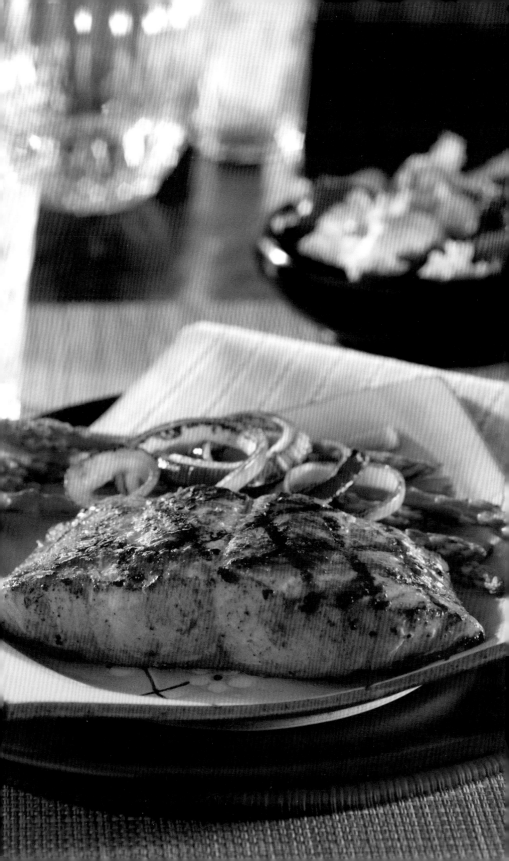

Lemon-Garlic Salmon with Tzaziki Sauce

½ cup diced cucumber
¾ teaspoon salt, divided
1 cup plain nonfat Greek yogurt
2 tablespoons lemon juice, divided
1 teaspoon grated lemon peel, divided
1 teaspoon minced garlic, divided
¼ teaspoon black pepper
4 skinless salmon fillets (about 4 ounces *each*)

1 Place cucumber in small colander set over small bowl; sprinkle with ¼ teaspoon salt. Drain 1 hour.

2 For Tzaziki Sauce, stir yogurt, cucumber, 1 tablespoon lemon juice, ½ teaspoon lemon peel, ½ teaspoon garlic and ¼ teaspoon salt in small bowl until combined. Cover and refrigerate until ready to use.

3 Combine remaining 1 tablespoon lemon juice, ½ teaspoon lemon peel, ½ teaspoon garlic, ¼ teaspoon salt and pepper in small bowl; mix well. Rub evenly onto salmon.

4 Heat nonstick grill pan over medium-high heat. Cook salmon 5 minutes per side or until fish begins to flake when tested with fork. Serve with Tzaziki Sauce.

Makes 4 servings

Serving Suggestion
Serve this Mediterranean-inspired dish with fresh vegetables or a savory salad, if desired.

nutrients per serving

Calories 243	**Total Fat** 12g	**Sodium** 508mg
Protein 29g	**Saturated Fat** 2g	**Fiber** 0g
Carbohydrate 3g	**Cholesterol** 60mg	

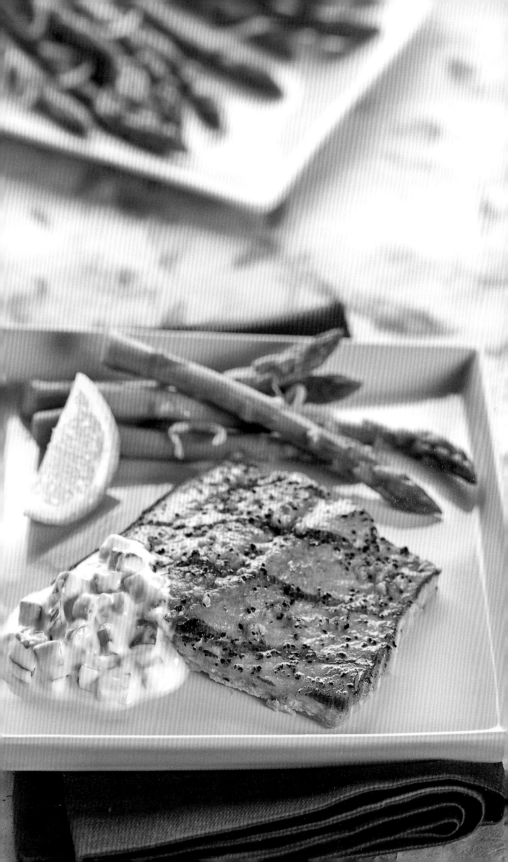

Baked Orange Roughy with Sautéed Vegetables

2 orange roughy fillets (about 4 ounces *each***)**
2 teaspoons olive oil
1 medium carrot, cut into matchstick-size pieces
4 medium mushrooms, sliced
⅓ cup chopped onion
¼ cup chopped green or yellow bell pepper
1 clove garlic, minced
Black pepper
Lemon wedges

1 Preheat oven to 350°F. Place fish fillets in shallow baking dish. Bake 15 minutes or until fish flakes easily when tested with fork.

2 Heat oil in small nonstick skillet over medium-high heat. Add carrot; cook 3 minutes, stirring occasionally. Add mushrooms, onion, bell pepper and garlic; cook and stir 2 minutes or until vegetables are crisp-tender.

3 Place fish on serving plates; top with vegetable mixture. Sprinkle with black pepper. Serve with lemon wedges.

Makes 2 servings

Notes

To microwave fish, place fish in shallow microwavable dish. Microwave, covered, on HIGH 2 minutes or until fish flakes easily when tested with fork.

To broil fish, place fish on rack of broiler pan. Broil 4 to 6 inches from heat 4 minutes on each side or until fish flakes easily when tested with fork.

nutrients per serving

Calories 157	**Total Fat** 6g	**Sodium** 84mg
Protein 18g	**Saturated Fat** 1g	**Fiber** 3g
Carbohydrate 10g	**Cholesterol** 22mg	

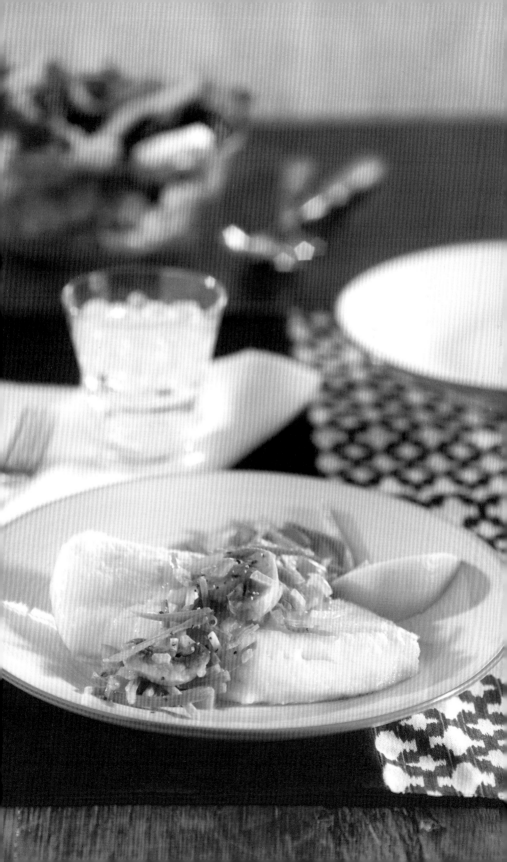

Skillet Shrimp over Couscous

½ **pound large raw shrimp, peeled and deveined**
3 **tablespoons lemon juice, divided**
⅛ **teaspoon plus ¼ teaspoon salt, divided**
¼ **teaspoon black pepper, divided**
2 **to 3 tablespoons chopped fresh Italian parsley**
1 **cup water**
⅔ **cup uncooked couscous**
1 **cup frozen peas, thawed**
3 **tablespoons thinly sliced green onion (white and light green parts)**
2 **teaspoons extra virgin olive oil**

1 Heat large skillet coated with nonstick cooking spray over medium-high heat. Add shrimp; cook 4 minutes or until pink and opaque. Remove from heat, add 2 tablespoons lemon juice, ⅛ teaspoon salt, ⅛ teaspoon pepper and parsley; toss to combine.

2 Meanwhile, to make couscous, bring water to a boil in a medium saucepan. Sprinkle couscous over top. Remove from heat and stir in peas, onion, oil, remaining ¼ teaspoon salt and ⅛ teaspoon pepper. Cover and let stand 5 minutes. Add remaining 1 tablespoon lemon juice; stir with a fork. Serve shrimp over couscous.

Makes 4 servings

nutrients per serving

Calories 232	**Total Fat** 4g	**Sodium** 336mg
Protein 18g	**Saturated Fat** 1g	**Fiber** 4g
Carbohydrate 32g	**Cholesterol** 86mg	

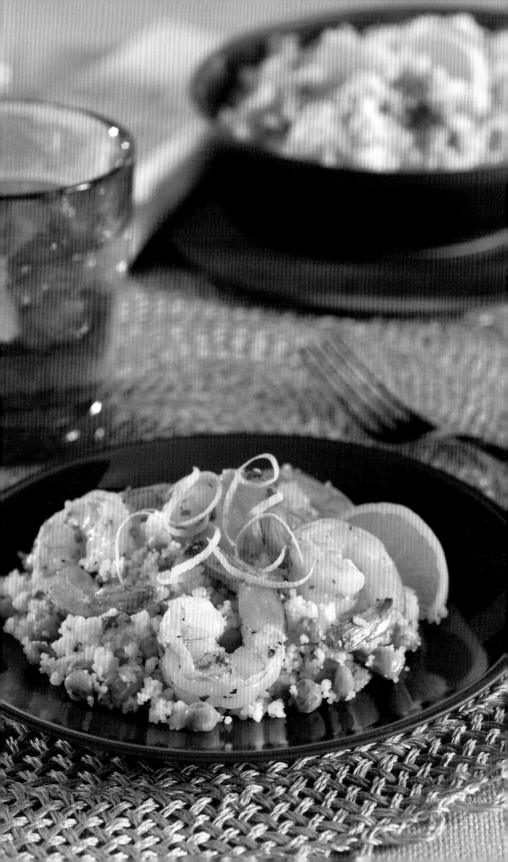

Tilapia & Sweet Corn Baked in Parchment

⅔ cup fresh or frozen corn
¼ cup finely chopped onion
¼ cup finely chopped red bell pepper
2 cloves garlic, minced
1 teaspoon chopped fresh rosemary leaves *or* ½ teaspoon dried rosemary, divided

½ teaspoon salt, divided
¼ to ½ teaspoon black pepper, divided
2 tilapia fillets (4 ounces *each*)
1 teaspoon olive oil

1 Preheat oven to 400°F. Cut two 15-inch squares of parchment paper; fold each piece in half.

2 Combine corn, onion, bell pepper, garlic, ½ teaspoon fresh rosemary, ¼ teaspoon salt and half the black pepper in small bowl. Open parchment paper; spoon half the corn mixture on one side of each piece, spreading out slightly.

3 Arrange tilapia fillets on top of corn mixture. Brush fish with oil; sprinkle with remaining ½ teaspoon fresh rosemary, ¼ teaspoon salt and black pepper.

4 To seal packets, fold other half of parchment over fish and corn. Fold and crimp along edges until completely sealed. Place packets on baking sheet.

5 Bake 15 minutes or until fish is opaque throughout. Remove packets to serving plates. Carefully cut centers of packets and peel back paper. Garnish as desired.

Makes 2 servings

Note
Heavy-duty foil can be substituted for the parchment paper. To serve, remove fish and corn from foil.

nutrients per serving

Calories 189
Protein 24g
Carbohydrate 15g

Total Fat 5g
Saturated Fat 1g
Cholesterol 0mg

Sodium 622mg
Fiber 2g

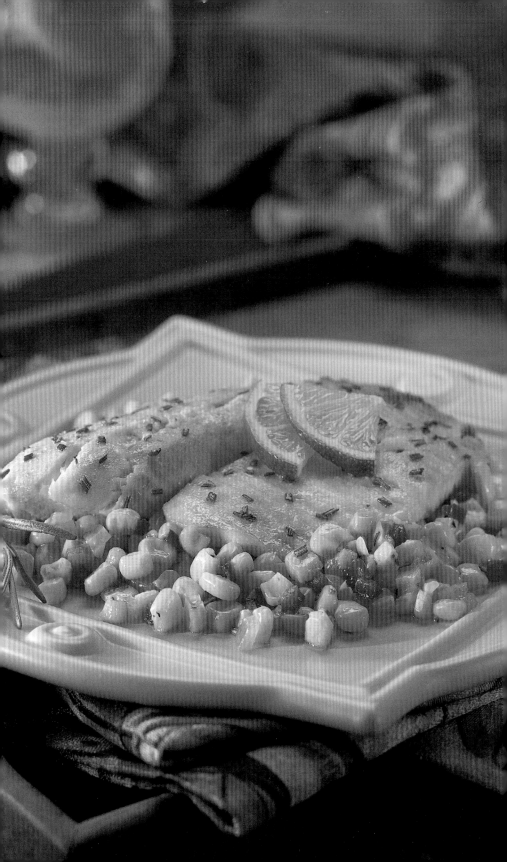

Baked Shrimp over Curried Tomatoes

2 teaspoons margarine, divided
1 small onion, finely chopped (½ cup)
4 medium tomatoes, seeded and chopped
½ to ¾ teaspoon curry powder
¼ teaspoon salt
⅛ teaspoon black pepper
⅛ teaspoon sugar (optional)
8 ounces jumbo raw shrimp, peeled, deveined and butterflied (8 shrimp)
1 slice potato bread or white whole wheat bread, cut into ½-inch cubes

1 Preheat oven to 400°F. Melt 1 teaspoon margarine in large nonstick skillet over medium-high heat. Add onion; cook 3 to 5 minutes or until tender. Add tomatoes, curry powder, salt and pepper; cook 2 to 3 minutes or until mixture is pulpy. Taste for sweetness and add sugar, if desired; cook 30 seconds.

2 Spoon mixture into 9-inch glass pie plate or large shallow baking dish. Top with shrimp and sprinkle with bread cubes. Melt remaining margarine in same skillet; drizzle over bread cubes.

3 Bake 10 to 14 minutes or until shrimp are pink and opaque.

Makes 2 servings (1¼ cups per serving)

nutrients per serving

Calories 251
Protein 27g
Carbohydrate 21g

Total Fat 7g
Saturated Fat 1g
Cholesterol 150mg

Sodium 606mg
Fiber 4g

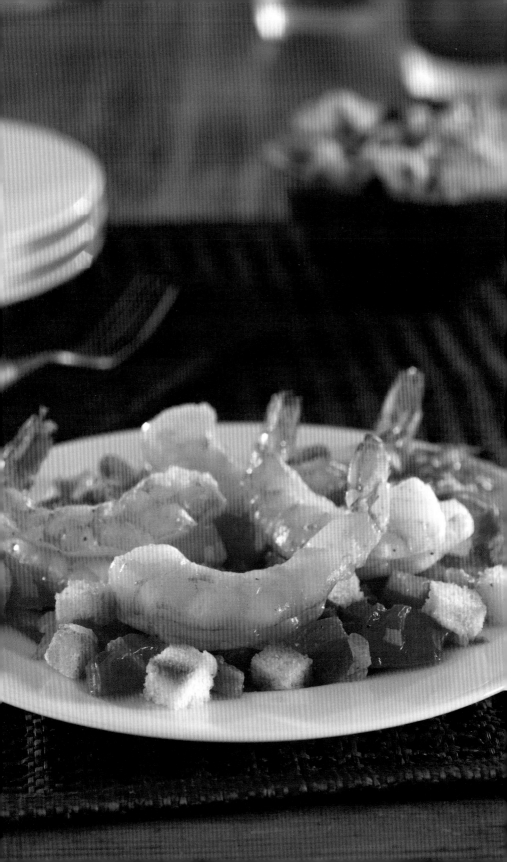

MEATLESS MEALS

Stuffed Squash with Black Beans

1 cup water, divided
1 acorn squash (2 pounds), quartered, seeded, skin pierced with fork
Salt and black pepper
⅓ cup pine nuts (1½ ounces)
1 cup chopped onion
1 medium red bell pepper, chopped
1 teaspoon ground cinnamon
¼ teaspoon ground allspice (optional)
1 cup canned black beans, rinsed and drained
¼ cup raisins
1 teaspoon sugar (optional)
¼ teaspoon salt
2 ounces crumbled goat or reduced-fat feta cheese (optional)

1 Pour ½ cup water into large microwavable dish. Place squash, skin side up, in dish. Sprinkle with salt and pepper. Cover with plastic wrap. Microwave on HIGH 12 minutes or until tender.

2 Meanwhile, heat medium nonstick skillet over medium-high heat. Add pine nuts; cook and stir 1 minute or until lightly browned. Remove to plate.

3 Spray skillet with nonstick cooking spray. Add onion and bell pepper; cook and stir 5 minutes or until vegetables just begin to brown. Add cinnamon and allspice, if desired; cook and stir 30 seconds. Add beans, raisins, sugar, if desired, and ¼ teaspoon salt. Stir in remaining ½ cup water. Remove from heat. Cover; let stand 2 minutes.

4 Place squash pieces on four serving plates. Spoon bean mixture in center of each squash piece. Sprinkle with pine nuts and cheese, if desired.

Makes 4 servings

nutrients per serving

Calories 223
Protein 6g
Carbohydrate 39g

Total Fat 8g
Saturated Fat 1g
Cholesterol 0mg

Sodium 356mg
Fiber 7g

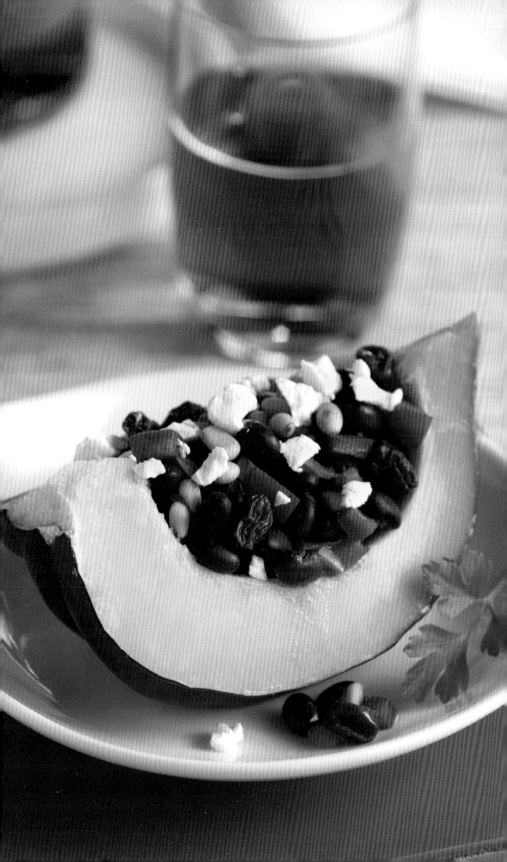

Vegetarian Paella

2 teaspoons canola oil
1 cup chopped onion
2 cloves garlic, minced
1 cup uncooked brown rice
2¼ cups vegetable broth
1 can (about 14½ ounces) no-salt-added stewed tomatoes
1 small zucchini, halved lengthwise and sliced to ½-inch thickness
    (about 1¼ cups)
1 cup chopped red bell pepper
2 teaspoons Italian seasoning
½ teaspoon ground turmeric
⅛ teaspoon ground red pepper
1 can (14 ounces) quartered artichoke hearts, drained
½ cup frozen baby peas
¾ teaspoon salt (optional)

Slow Cooker Directions

1 Heat oil in small nonstick skillet over medium-high heat. Add onion; cook and stir 6 to 7 minutes or until tender. Stir in garlic. Transfer to slow cooker. Stir in rice.

2 Add broth, tomatoes, zucchini, bell pepper, Italian seasoning, turmeric and red pepper; mix well. Cover; cook on LOW 4 hours or on HIGH 2 hours or until liquid is absorbed.

3 Stir in artichokes, peas and salt, if desired. Cover; cook 5 to 10 minutes or until vegetables are tender.

Makes 6 servings (about 1½ cups per serving)

nutrients per serving

Calories 241
Protein 5g
Carbohydrate 43g

Total Fat 7g
Saturated Fat 1g
Cholesterol 0mg

Sodium 470mg
Fiber 7g

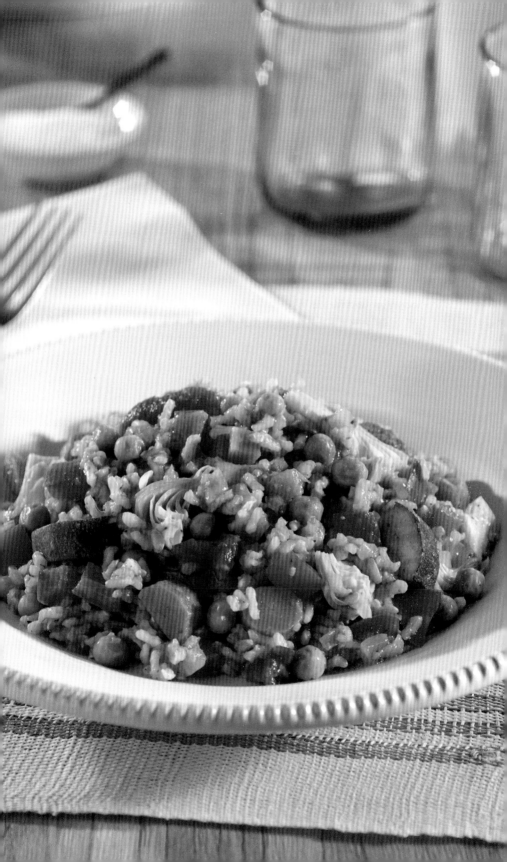

Veggie Tostadas

1 tablespoon olive oil
1 cup chopped onion
1 cup chopped celery
2 cloves garlic, chopped
1 can (about 15 ounces) red kidney beans, rinsed and drained
1 can (about 15 ounces) Great Northern beans, rinsed and drained
1 can (about 14 ounces) salsa-style diced tomatoes
2 teaspoons mild chili powder
1 teaspoon ground cumin
6 (6-inch) corn tortillas
    Toppings: chopped fresh cilantro, shredded lettuce, chopped seeded fresh tomatoes, shredded reduced-fat Cheddar cheese and fat-free sour cream (optional)

1 Heat oil in large skillet over medium heat. Add onion, celery and garlic. Cook and stir 8 minutes or until softened. Add beans and tomatoes. Stir to blend. Add chili powder and cumin; stir. Reduce heat to medium-low. Simmer 30 minutes, stirring occasionally, until thickened.

2 Meanwhile, preheat oven to 400°F. Place tortillas in single layer directly on oven rack. Bake 10 to 12 minutes or until crisp. Place one tortilla on each plate. Spoon bean mixture evenly over each tortilla. Top with cilantro, lettuce, tomatoes, Cheddar cheese and sour cream, if desired.

Makes 6 servings (1 tortilla with ⅔ cup bean mixture per serving)

nutrients per serving

Calories 208
Protein 10g
Carbohydrate 39g
Total Fat 3g
Saturated Fat 1g
Cholesterol 0mg
Sodium 945mg
Fiber 10g

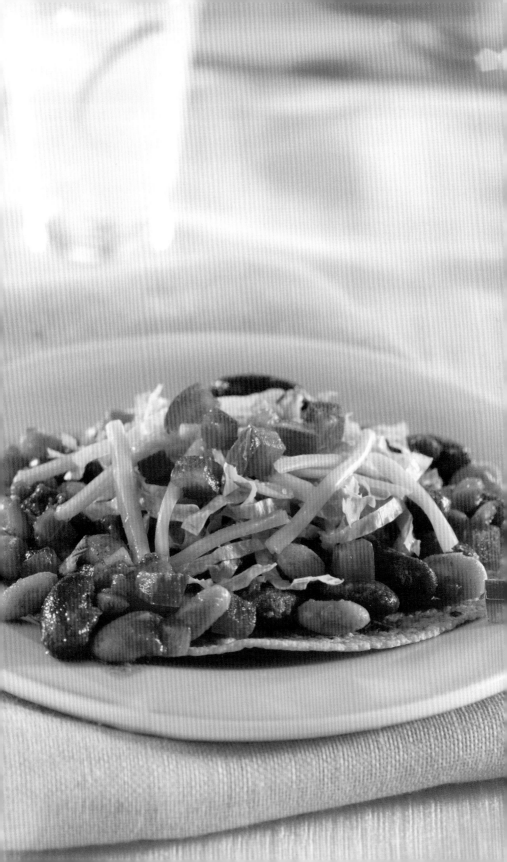

Quinoa & Vegetable Medley

Nonstick cooking spray
2 medium sweet potatoes, cut into ½-inch-thick slices
1 medium eggplant, peeled and cut into ½-inch cubes
1 medium tomato, cut into wedges
1 large green bell pepper, sliced
1 small onion, cut into wedges
½ teaspoon salt
¼ teaspoon black pepper
¼ teaspoon ground red pepper
1 cup uncooked quinoa
2 cloves garlic, minced
½ teaspoon dried thyme
¼ teaspoon dried marjoram
2 cups water or fat-free reduced-sodium vegetable broth

Slow Cooker Directions

1 Coat slow cooker with nonstick cooking spray. Combine sweet potatoes, eggplant, tomato, bell pepper and onion and toss with salt, black pepper and red pepper in slow cooker.

2 Meanwhile, place quinoa in strainer; rinse well. Add to vegetable mixture. Stir in garlic, thyme, marjoram and broth. Cover; cook on LOW 5 hours or on HIGH 2½ hours or until quinoa is tender and broth is absorbed.

Makes 6 servings (1¼ cups per serving)

nutrients per serving

Calories 193
Protein 6g
Carbohydrate 40g
Total Fat 2g
Saturated Fat 1g
Cholesterol 0mg
Sodium 194mg
Fiber 6g

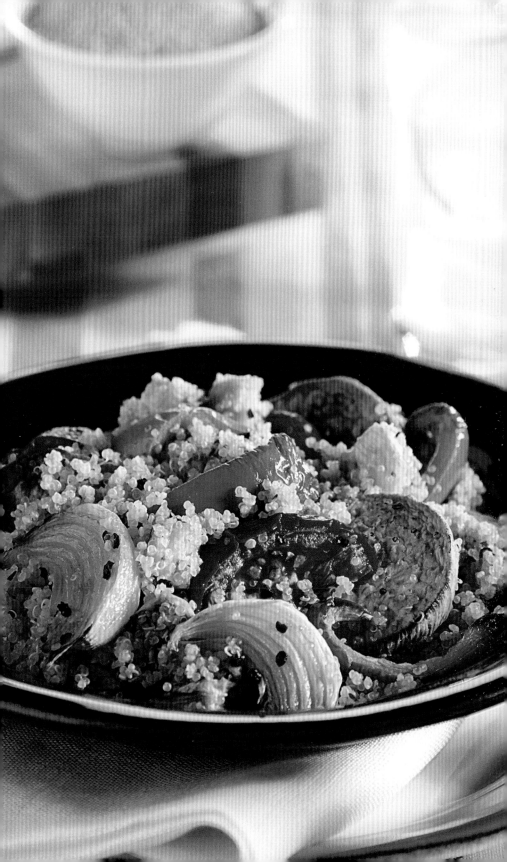

Spaghetti and Vegetable Frittata

Nonstick cooking spray
1 package (8 ounces) sliced mushrooms
1 cup thinly sliced leeks (white and light green parts)
5 egg whites
1 whole egg
⅓ cup fat-free (skim) milk
3 tablespoons grated Parmesan cheese
⅛ teaspoon ground nutmeg
¼ teaspoon salt
⅛ teaspoon black pepper
1 package (10 ounces) frozen chopped collards, thawed and squeezed dry
2 cups cooked whole grain spaghetti
½ cup (2 ounces) shredded part-skim mozzarella cheese

1 Spray large ovenproof skillet with nonstick cooking spray; heat over medium-high heat. Add mushrooms and leeks; cook and stir 8 minutes or until lightly browned.

2 Whisk egg whites, whole egg, milk, Parmesan cheese, nutmeg, salt and pepper in large bowl. Stir in collards, spaghetti and mushroom mixture. Coat same skillet with cooking spray; heat over medium-low heat. Add egg mixture; cover and cook 10 minutes or until top is set.

3 Meanwhile, preheat broiler. Sprinkle mozzarella cheese over frittata; broil about 5 inches from heat 3 minutes or until golden brown. Cut into six wedges.

Makes 6 servings

nutrients per serving

Calories 156	**Total Fat** 4g	**Sodium** 285mg
Protein 13g	**Saturated Fat** 2g	**Fiber** 4g
Carbohydrate 20g	**Cholesterol** 39mg	

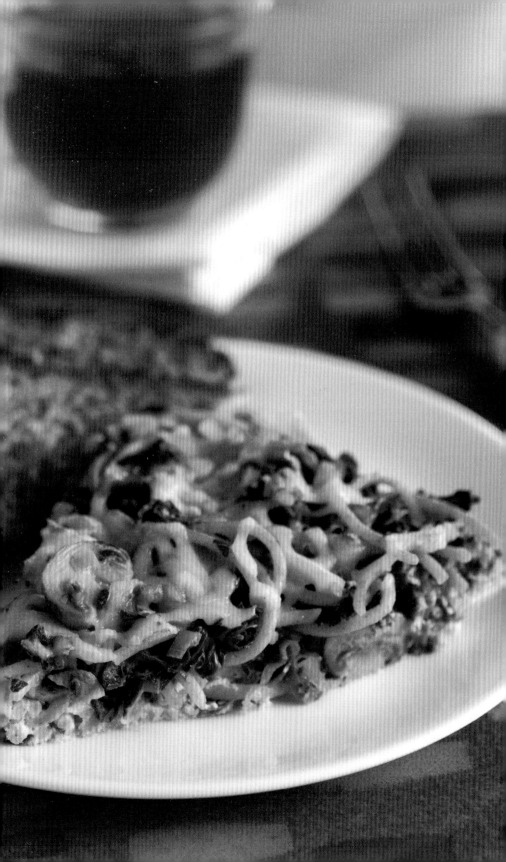

Veggie "Meatballs"

½ cup water
¾ cup bulgur wheat
2 teaspoons olive oil
3 medium portobello mushrooms (10 ounces), stemmed and diced
1 small onion, chopped
1 small zucchini (6 ounces), coarsely grated
1 teaspoon Italian seasoning
2 cloves garlic, minced
¼ cup sun-dried tomatoes (not packed in oil*), chopped
4 ounces grated Parmesan cheese
2 egg whites
2 cups low-fat marinara sauce, heated

If unavailable you may substitute ¼ cup sun-dried tomatoes packed in oil, well drained, patted dry and chopped.

1 Preheat oven to 375°F. Line large rimmed baking sheet with foil; spray with nonstick cooking spray.

2 Bring water to a boil in small saucepan; remove from heat. Stir in bulgur; cover and let stand while preparing vegetables.

3 Heat oil in large nonstick skillet over medium-high heat. Add mushrooms, onion, zucchini and Italian seasoning; cook and stir about 8 minutes or until softened. Add garlic; cook and stir 1 minute. Stir in tomatoes.

4 Transfer mushroom mixture to large bowl; let cool slightly. Add bulgur, Parmesan cheese and egg whites; mix well. Shape mixture into 12 balls using ¼ cup for each. Place meatballs on prepared baking sheet.

5 Bake 20 minutes. Turn meatballs; bake 8 to 10 minutes or until well browned. Serve hot with marinara sauce.

Makes 4 servings (3 "meatballs" and ½ cup sauce per serving)

nutrients per serving

Calories 280
Protein 18g
Carbohydrate 32g

Total Fat 10g
Saturated Fat 3g
Cholesterol 18mg

Sodium 510mg
Fiber 8g

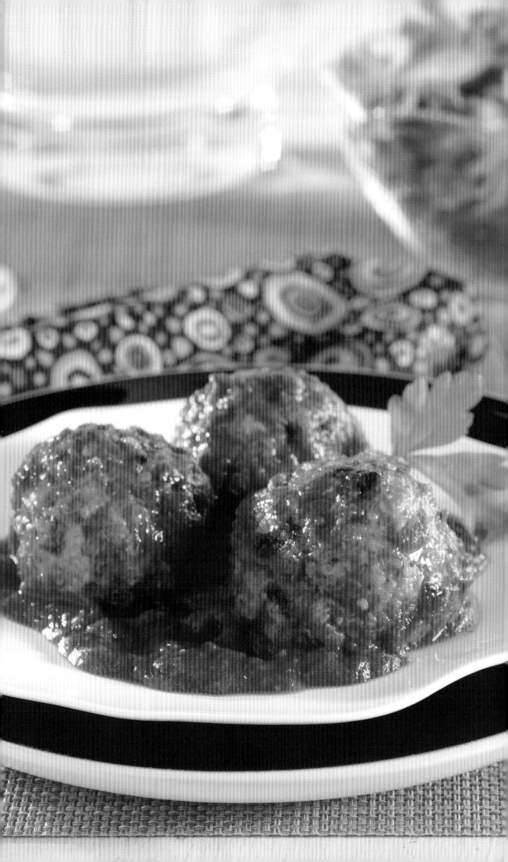

Roasted Beet Risotto

2 medium beets, trimmed
1 container (32 ounces) low-sodium vegetable broth, divided
1 tablespoon canola oil
1 cup uncooked Arborio rice
1 medium leek, white and light green parts only, finely chopped
½ cup crumbled goat cheese, plus additional for garnish
1 teaspoon Italian seasoning
¼ teaspoon salt
    Juice of 1 lemon
    Lemon wedges (optional)

1 Preheat oven to 400°F. Wrap each beet tightly in foil. Place on baking sheet. Roast 45 minutes to 1 hour or until knife inserted into centers goes in easily. Unwrap beets; discard foil. Let stand 15 minutes or until cool enough to handle. Peel and cut beets into bite-size pieces. Set aside.

2 Heat broth to a simmer in medium saucepan; keep warm.

3 Heat oil in separate medium saucepan over medium-high heat. Add rice; cook and stir 1 to 2 minutes. Add leek; cook and stir 1 to 2 minutes. Add broth, ½ cup at a time, stirring constantly until broth is absorbed before adding next ½ cup. Continue adding broth and stirring until rice is tender and mixture is creamy, about 20 to 25 minutes. Remove from heat.

4 Stir ½ cup cheese, Italian seasoning and salt into risotto. Gently stir in beets. Sprinkle with lemon juice and additional cheese, if desired. Garnish with lemon wedges. Serve immediately.

Makes 4 servings (about ¾ cup per serving)

nutrients per serving

Calories 278	Total Fat 8g	Sodium 383mg
Protein 8g	Saturated Fat 3g	Fiber 2g
Carbohydrate 45g	Cholesterol 9mg	

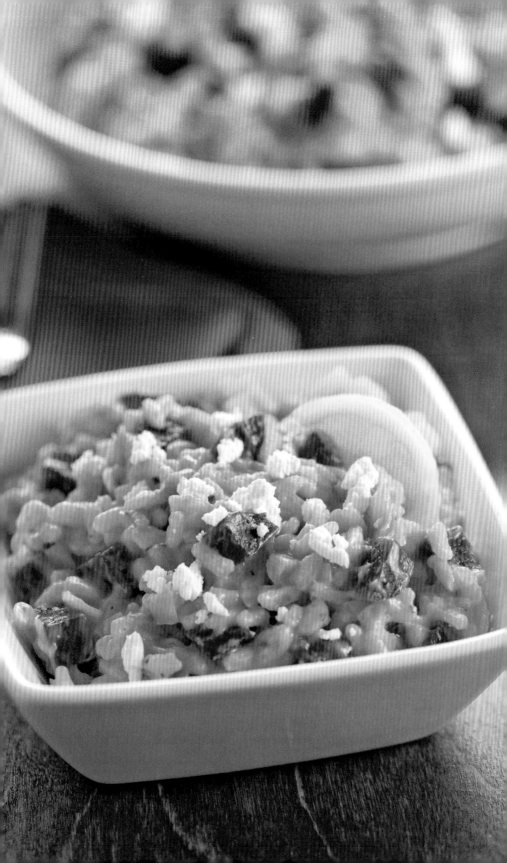

Vegetarian Jambalaya

1 tablespoon vegetable oil
½ cup diced green or red bell pepper
1 can (about 14 ounces) diced tomatoes with chiles
1 package (12 ounces) ground taco/burrito flavor soy meat substitute, crumbled
1 package (about 9 ounces) New Orleans style ready-to-serve jambalaya rice
2 tablespoons water

1 Heat oil in large skillet over medium-high heat. Add bell pepper; cook and stir 3 minutes.

2 Add tomatoes, soy crumbles and rice; mix well. Stir in water. Cook 5 minutes, uncovered, or until heated through.

Makes 4 servings

nutrients per serving

Calories 281
Protein 12g
Carbohydrate 49g

Total Fat 4g
Saturated Fat 1g
Cholesterol 0mg

Sodium 1012mg
Fiber 4g

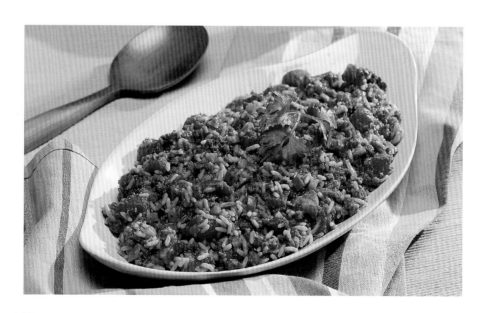

Vegetarian Stir Fry

1 package (12.3 ounces) firm tofu
½ tablespoon salt-free seasoning blend
½ cup uncooked instant brown rice
1 bag (12 ounces) ready-to-use vegetable stir-fry mix
½ cup low-fat sesame ginger salad dressing

1 Preheat indoor covered grill per grill instructions. Cut tofu into four (1-inch) slices. Sprinkle slices with seasoning blend. Grill for 5 to 6 minutes. Set aside.

2 Prepare rice according to package instructions, omitting salt and fat. Cook vegetables in microwave according to package instructions. Toss vegetables with dressing in mixing bowl. Divide vegetables among four plates. Top with tofu slice.

Makes 4 servings

Tip
Serve with orange segments and pineapple chunks.

nutrients per serving

Calories 239
Protein 10g
Carbohydrate 23g

Total Fat 11g
Saturated Fat 1g
Cholesterol 0mg

Sodium 245mg
Fiber 2g

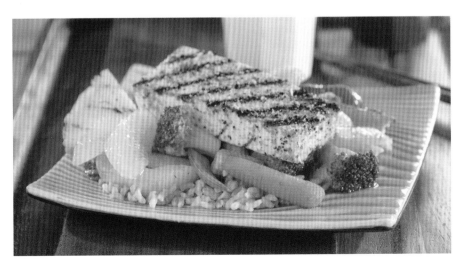

Quinoa Burrito Bowls

1 cup uncooked quinoa
2 cups water
2 tablespoons fresh lime juice, divided
¼ cup light sour cream
2 teaspoons vegetable oil
1 small onion, diced
1 red bell pepper, diced
1 clove garlic, minced
½ cup canned black beans, rinsed and drained
½ cup thawed frozen corn
Shredded lettuce
Lime wedges (optional)

1 Place quinoa in fine-mesh strainer; rinse well under cold running water. Bring 2 cups water to a boil in small saucepan; stir in quinoa. Reduce heat to low; cover and simmer 10 to 15 minutes or until quinoa is tender and water is absorbed. Stir in 1 tablespoon lime juice. Cover and keep warm. Combine sour cream and remaining 1 tablespoon lime juice; set aside.

2 Meanwhile, heat oil in large skillet over medium heat. Add onion and bell pepper; cook and stir 5 minutes or until softened. Add garlic; cook 1 minute. Add black beans and corn; cook 3 to 5 minutes or until heated through.

3 Divide quinoa among four serving bowls; top with black bean mixture, lettuce and sour cream mixture. Garnish with lime wedges.

Makes 4 servings

nutrients per serving

Calories 258
Protein 9g
Carbohydrate 42g
Total Fat 7g
Saturated Fat 1g
Cholesterol 4mg
Sodium 136mg
Fiber 6g

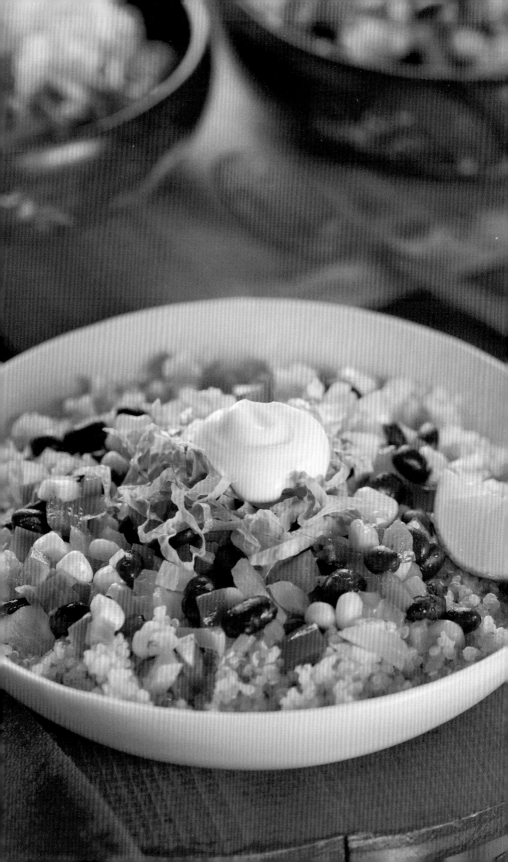

Eggplant Parmesan

2 egg whites
2 tablespoons water
6 tablespoons Italian-seasoned dry bread crumbs
2 tablespoons grated Parmesan cheese plus ¼ cup grated Parmesan cheese, divided
1 large eggplant, peeled and cut into 12 round slices
2 teaspoons olive oil
1 small onion, diced
1 clove garlic, minced
2 cans (about 14 ounces each) no-salt-added diced tomatoes
½ teaspoon dried basil
½ teaspoon dried oregano
½ cup (2 ounces) shredded part-skim mozzarella cheese

1 Preheat oven to 350°F. Spray 15×10×1-inch jelly-roll pan with nonstick cooking spray.

2 Whisk egg whites and water in shallow dish. Combine bread crumbs and 2 tablespoons Parmesan cheese in another shallow dish. Dip eggplant slices in egg white mixture, then in bread crumb mixture, pressing lightly to adhere crumbs.

3 Place eggplant slices in single layer in prepared pan. Bake 25 to 30 minutes or until bottoms are browned. Turn slices; bake 15 to 20 minutes or until well browned and tender.

4 Meanwhile, heat oil in medium nonstick skillet over medium-high heat. Add onion; cook and stir 5 minutes or until softened. Add garlic; cook and stir 1 minute. Stir in tomatoes, basil and oregano; bring to a boil. Reduce heat to low; simmer 15 to 20 minutes or until sauce is thickened, stirring occasionally.

5 Spray 13×9-inch baking dish with cooking spray. Spread sauce in dish. Arrange eggplant slices in single layer on top of sauce. Sprinkle with mozzarella cheese and ¼ cup Parmesan cheese. Bake 15 to 20 minutes or until sauce is bubbly and cheese melts.

Makes 4 servings

nutrients per serving

Calories 227	**Total Fat** 8g	**Sodium** 610mg
Protein 12g	**Saturated Fat** 2g	**Fiber** 9g
Carbohydrate 31g	**Cholesterol** 11mg	

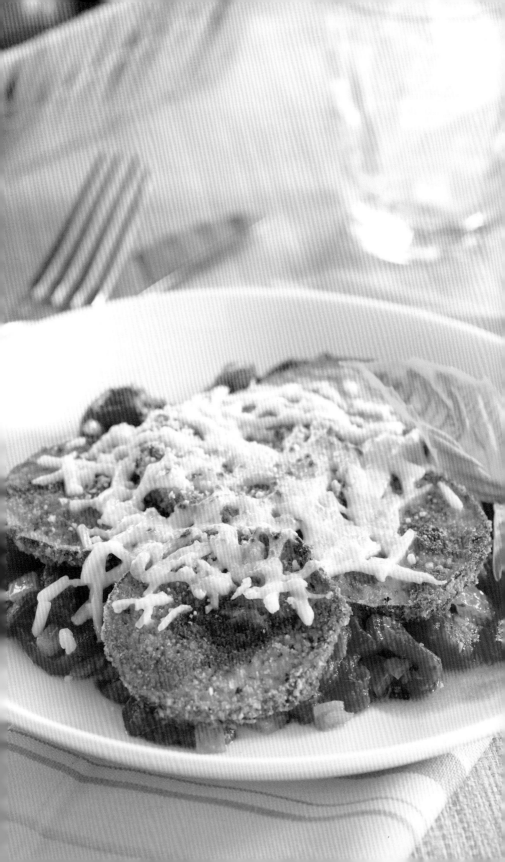

INDEX

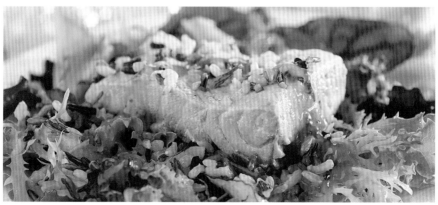

METRIC CONVERSION CHART

VOLUME MEASUREMENTS (dry)

$^1/_8$ teaspoon = 0.5 mL
$^1/_4$ teaspoon = 1 mL
$^1/_2$ teaspoon = 2 mL
$^3/_4$ teaspoon = 4 mL
1 teaspoon = 5 mL
1 tablespoon = 15 mL
2 tablespoons = 30 mL
$^1/_4$ cup = 60 mL
$^1/_3$ cup = 75 mL
$^1/_2$ cup = 125 mL
$^2/_3$ cup = 150 mL
$^3/_4$ cup = 175 mL
1 cup = 250 mL
2 cups = 1 pint = 500 mL
3 cups = 750 mL
4 cups = 1 quart = 1 L

VOLUME MEASUREMENTS (fluid)

1 fluid ounce (2 tablespoons) = 30 mL
4 fluid ounces ($^1/_2$ cup) = 125 mL
8 fluid ounces (1 cup) = 250 mL
12 fluid ounces (1$^1/_2$ cups) = 375 mL
16 fluid ounces (2 cups) = 500 mL

WEIGHTS (mass)

$^1/_2$ ounce = 15 g
1 ounce = 30 g
3 ounces = 90 g
4 ounces = 120 g
8 ounces = 225 g
10 ounces = 285 g
12 ounces = 360 g
16 ounces = 1 pound = 450 g

DIMENSIONS

$^1/_{16}$ inch = 2 mm
$^1/_8$ inch = 3 mm
$^1/_4$ inch = 6 mm
$^1/_2$ inch = 1.5 cm
$^3/_4$ inch = 2 cm
1 inch = 2.5 cm

OVEN TEMPERATURES

250°F = 120°C
275°F = 140°C
300°F = 150°C
325°F = 160°C
350°F = 180°C
375°F = 190°C
400°F = 200°C
425°F = 220°C
450°F = 230°C

BAKING PAN SIZES

Utensil	Size in Inches/Quarts	Metric Volume	Size in Centimeters
Baking or	8×8×2	2 L	20×20×5
Cake Pan	9×9×2	2.5 L	23×23×5
(square or	12×8×2	3 L	30×20×5
rectangular)	13×9×2	3.5 L	33×23×5
Loaf Pan	8×4×3	1.5 L	20×10×7
	9×5×3	2 L	23×13×7
Round Layer	8×1½	1.2 L	20×4
Cake Pan	9×1½	1.5 L	23×4
Pie Plate	8×1¼	750 mL	20×3
	9×1¼	1 L	23×3
Baking Dish	1 quart	1 L	—
or Casserole	1½ quart	1.5 L	—
	2 quart	2 L	—